All I Want Is a
Good Night's Sleep

All I Want Is a Good Night's Sleep

SONIA ANCOLI-ISRAEL, PhD

Professor, Department of Psychiatry,
University of California, San Diego, School of Medicine
Director, Sleep Disorders Clinic,
Veterans Affairs Medical Center, San Diego

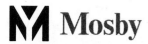 Mosby

St. Louis   Baltimore   Boston   Carlsbad   Chicago   Naples   New York   Philadelphia   Portland
London   Madrid   Mexico City   Singapore   Sydney   Tokyo   Toronto   Wiesbaden

Vice President and Publisher: Don Ladig
Editor: Jennifer Roche
Developmental Editor: Anne Gleason
Project Manager: Patricia Tannian
Production Editor: Melissa Mraz
Composition Specialist: Terri Bovay
Book Design Manager: Gail Morey Hudson
Manufacturing Manager: Dave Graybill
Cover Design: Teresa Breckwoldt

Printed in the United States of America
Composition by Mosby Electronic Production
Printing/binding by Plus Communications

Mosby–Year Book, Inc.
11830 Westline Industrial Drive
St. Louis, Missouri 63146

Library of Congress Cataloging in Publication Data

Ancoli-Israel, Sonia.
    All I want is a good night's sleep / Sonia Ancoli-Israel.
        p.   cm.
    Includes bibliographical references.
    ISBN 0-8151-4843-7
    1. Sleep disorders—Popular works. I. Title.
RC547.A58 1996
616.8'498—dc20   96-201
                                                                          CIP

96 97 98 99 00 / 9 8 7 6 5 4 3 2 1

To my father

Nissan Ancoli

who went to sleep for a final time
but will always be awake in my heart.

About the Author

Dr. Sonia Ancoli-Israel received her Ph.D. in Psychology from the University of California, San Francisco. Dr. Ancoli-Israel is a professor in the Department of Psychiatry at the University of California, San Diego, and is Director of the Sleep Disorders Clinic at the San Diego Veterans Affairs Medical Center. She is widely recognized as one of the world's leading authorities in the area of sleep in the elderly.

She has over 200 scientific publications and has been a member of the Board of Directors of the Sleep Research Society, the National Sleep Foundation, Association for Applied Psychophysiology and Biofeedback, and the Society for Light Treatment and Biological Rhythms.

Foreword

"Turn out the lights, the party's over!" This refrain is an excellent metaphor for the modern American's approach to sleep—that is, sleep simply is not an option until all the fun, furor, and feverish activities of the day are finished. As a consequence of increasingly hectic lifestyles, sleep has somehow become a lost commodity—lost and relegated to a nuisance that must be tolerated rather than a fundamental component of a healthy life. Sleep is an afterthought in today's fast-forward lifestyle. Thus, beyond a handful of scientists and clinicians, the people most concerned with sleep are those who cannot attain it or for whom even an overabundance of sleep is insufficient.

More has been learned about sleep and sleep disorders in the last 25 years than in all of preceding human history, and most of this knowledge resulted from research supported by the National Institutes of Health. Sadly, little of this information has been communicated to the public at large. The National Commission on Sleep Disorders Research recently held a series of hearings in many parts of the country, and time and again people from all walks of life testified on how they were confronted by—as Senator Mark Hatfield so aptly put it—vast reservoirs of ignorance about sleep and sleep disorders. Not surprisingly, two of the Commission's final recommendations focused on education: one urged support for training of health care professionals and the second recommended "that a major public awareness/education campaign about sleep and sleep disorders be undertaken immediately by the Federal Government."*

All I Want Is a Good Night's Sleep fills many of the knowledge gaps. Dr. Ancoli-Israel's book provides an easily accessible gateway to the essential nature of sleep and to the components of sleep that can fail and cause great discomfort. She has accomplished in these pages the difficult task of making esoteric facts about sleep comprehensible to nonscientists, and her easygoing style brings the reader closer to understanding principles of good sleep hygiene, what can go wrong with sleep, and suggestions on how to improve sleep. This book represents an outstanding beginning in the effort to fill the "reservoir of ignorance" with knowledge. By uncloaking some of sleep's many mysteries, this book may be particularly useful to those challenged by sleep disorders.

Thus I hope that all who read Dr. Ancoli-Israel's book will find and enjoy that sought after good night's sleep.

Mary A. Carskadon, PhD

Professor, Psychiatry and Human Behavior,
Brown University School of Medicine
Director of Chronobiology and Sleep Research,
E.P. Bradley Hospital
Member, National Commission on Sleep Disorders Research

Wake Up America: A National Sleep Alert. Executive Summary and Executive Report of the National Commission on Sleep Disorders Research, submitted to the United States Congress and to the Secretary, U.S. Department of Health and Human Services, January, 1993, p. vii.

Preface

Whenever I tell people that I study and work with individuals who have sleep disorders, I get one of two reactions. They say, "Oh, I sleep like a log. In fact, I could sleep standing up." Others sneer and declare, "Send your patients to me. I'll make them work hard for a day, and they won't have any trouble sleeping after that." What these comments tell *me* is that sleep disorders and sleep in general are widely misunderstood. "Sleeping standing up" may in fact indicate a problem with excessive sleepiness. Thinking that hard work will solve all insomnia problems is to deny that insomnia is real and can be brought about by serious problems.

These kinds of misconceptions led me to write this book. My purpose is to educate you—the person who has trouble sleeping—so that you will be able to understand the reasons behind the sleep problem and learn what you can do about it. We all know the mental and physical toll that even one sleepless night can take. Reading this book will help you begin to help yourself or a family member sleep better, and ultimately, feel better.

Sonia Ancoli-Israel

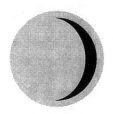 # Acknowledgments

I have many people to thank for their help in completing this book. Without each of them, the book would not have happened. Dr. Jack Clausen came to me with the idea of my writing this book and pointed Mosby in my direction. As a pulmonary physician, Dr. Clausen also helped write the chapter on sleep disordered breathing. Timothy V. Coy, one of my graduate students, helped write the first draft of chapters on narcolepsy and sleep of children. Annie Gilbar (my closest friend, my sister, and a professional writer), Dr. Mary Carskadon (a great friend and colleague who has always been an inspiration to me), and Melissa Bartell and Brenda Mann (two close friends who have nothing to do with the field of sleep) all read earlier drafts to assure me that I was headed on the right course. Dr. Carskadon even made time in her incredibly busy schedule to write the foreword to the book. Dr. Ruth Pat-Horenczyk (a new friend and colleague) read an earlier version and correctly made additions, particularly to the insomnia chapter, her area of expertise. Others who read the manuscript and supplied me with helpful comments were Marilyn Lewis, my colleague in arms who always keeps me sane, William Mason, who has worked with me longer than I care to remember, and my students Nayer Khazeni and Jennifer Martin. I would also like to thank my other research associates Carl Stepnowsky, Robert Fell, Denise Williams Jones, Sam Messin, and Charles Senger, and some of my more recent students, Dr. Camilla Clark, Einat Estline, Rena Kramer, Dr. Clete Kushida, Dr. Roberta (Bobbie) Lovell, Dr. Mary Moffit, and Dr. Rachel Morehouse. You taught me as much as I taught you. I also want to thank all my patients who taught me about sleep problems as I was helping them deal with theirs.

In a field as small as ours, there are many other friends and colleagues with whom I have worked over the years in one capacity or another and who, in one way or another, have helped me. I would have loved to thank each of you by name, but there are just too many of you. Thank you to my colleagues in San Diego, at the National Sleep Foundation, and in APSS and those others who also study sleep and aging. You have been part of the reason it has been so much fun to study sleep.

Because of the nature of this book, results of many research studies are cited without giving credit to the authors. Please forgive me as I could not overwhelm the reader with all the scientific references. But the reader should understand that it is the work of a multitude of fine sleep scientists and clinicians that has moved our field forward. It is also important for the reader to understand that the majority of the work that has led to our knowledge has been funded by the National Institutes of Health (including the National Institute of Aging, the National Institute of Mental Health, and the National Heart, Lung, and Blood Institute). Much of the work was done with humans, but much of our knowledge is also gleaned from animal research, without which we would never have the answers for some of the questions about problems of sleep.

I also want to thank James Shanahan, who first approached Jack Clausen and me about writing this book, Anne Gleason, who worked with me patiently as I learned what it means to write a book, Jan Ruvido, who did all the wonderful illustrations, and Nadine Sokol, who drew the graphs.

Most of all, I thank my family: my husband Andy, our children Sarah and David, my mother Esther Ancoli Barbasch, Arnold Israel, and Mark Barbasch, who have always been most loving, most patient, and most supportive and are the reason behind everything I do. You make the day worth waking up for.

Sonia Ancoli-Israel

Contents

1 Introduction, 1

2 What is Sleep? 3

3 Insomnia: Why Can't I Sleep? 15

4 Hypersomnia: Why Do I Sleep So Much? 31

5 Sleep Disordered Breathing, 35

6 Narcolepsy, 53

7 Periodic Limb Movements in Sleep, 61

8 Circadian Rhythms, 69

9 Sleep of Children, 81

10 Parasomnias, 91

11 Aging and Sleep, 101

12 Doctors, Drugs, and Devices, 109

Glossary, 127

Bibliography, 131

1 INTRODUCTION

Have you ever had a really bad night's sleep? You know, a night when you toss and turn, and you can't seem to get comfortable no matter how many times you fluff your pillow or try a different body position. A kind of night when you finally fall asleep just a few hours before your alarm clock goes off and wakes you right back up again.

Or are you the kind of person who has no trouble falling asleep, but a few hours later, there you are, wide awake? Of course, the first thing you do when you wake up in the middle of the night is what? You look at the clock! What difference does it make if it is 2:00 AM or 3:00 AM? Either way, you want to be asleep, not awake, right? And then you begin to toss and turn and fidget, and you make yourself so tense that you'll never be able to get back to sleep.

Do you find yourself relying on alcohol or pills to help you sleep? Are you taking so many different medications that you're not sure what they are doing to your sleep pattern? Do you have medical problems that also might be contributing to trouble with sleep?

Or perhaps you are the type of person who sleeps great at night, but during the day, you are still sleepy. Your co-workers are beginning to wonder what you really do at night, because there you are at your desk, or at a meeting, fighting to keep your eyes open. It seems all you want to do is sleep. Your wife (or husband) is complaining that you sleep too much, and you don't understand why you are so sleepy.

1

Does your family complain that you snore so loudly that they are threatening to move out, or worse, throw you out?

Maybe the one with the sleep problem is not you but your child. Is he walking during sleep? Banging into doors, setting off the alarm as he leaves the house in his sleep? Is your child wetting the bed at an age you think she should be dry?

Is your parent the one with the sleep problem? Is Grandma getting night and day confused—up at night and sleeping during the day?

All these complaints are symptoms of sleep disorders. Each chapter in this book addresses specific issues and tries to explain them to you—in English, not in medicalese—and gives you suggestions as to what can be done to help you. You can read the whole book or find the chapter that best fits your problem. Either way, the answers you find within these pages will help you get that "good night's sleep."

2) WHAT IS SLEEP?

Almost all people spend one third of their lives sleeping. Many people think of sleep as the opposite of being awake; our brain is energetic during wake and idle during sleep. In fact, sleep is a very active process that is controlled by specific parts of the brain. We go to sleep because certain parts of the brain, such as the basal forebrain, the thalamus, and the hypothalamus, have *increased* activity.

Sleep is part of a 24-hour cycle of activity and inactivity. What we do during the day affects how we sleep at night, and how we sleep at night affects how we feel during the day. This is called the homeostatic regulation of sleep. The longer you are awake, the more sleep you need. The more you sleep, the longer you can stay awake. Sleep therefore has a homeostatic function by reversing the feeling of sleepiness. The need to sleep builds up during the waking state and disappears during sleep.

Although we all sleep, the true purpose of sleep is still unknown. We do know that sleep is necessary—we can't do without it. We sleep when our bodies get very tired. If we do not sleep, our bodies are unable to function correctly. The longest anyone has ever been sleep deprived is 11 days. People who are severely sleep deprived have great difficulty staying awake during the day. Studies have shown that rats who are sleep deprived for about a month die. Some people believe that the purpose of sleep is to conserve or restore energy to parts of our body. Yet as we shall see, our bodies are quite active during sleep.

The second reason we sleep has to do with our biologic clocks, or circadian (Greek for "about [circa] a day [dies]") rhythms. Our biologic clocks are controlled by a part of the brain called the suprachiasmatic nucleus (SCN) (Fig. 2-1). The SCN in turn is controlled by exposure to light. For that reason we tend to sleep when it is dark and to be alert when it is light. In fact, we get sleepy at certain times because our circadian rhythms vary at distinct times. For example, most of us get sleepy in the late afternoon (when many societies take "siestas" and others feel what has been called the postprandial [after lunch] dip) and at night. This happens because our body temperature drops at those times. When our body temperature begins to drop, we are sleepier than when it begins to rise.

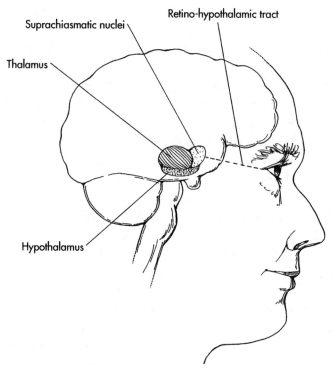

Fig. 2-1 Diagram of the brain.

Nearly all systems within our bodies cycle, including hormones and body temperature. When our rhythms get out of sync, such as with jet lag, our sleep becomes disturbed.

Although we do not know the real purpose of sleep, we do know that it is crucial for life. If we went without any sleep at all for several nights, we would not be able to function in our everyday lives.

HOW IS SLEEP MEASURED?

To study and observe the physiology of sleep, we use special equipment to record brain waves (electroencephalogram or EEG), eye movements (electrooculogram or EOG), and chin muscle tension (electromyogram or EMG), since these are the three variables that

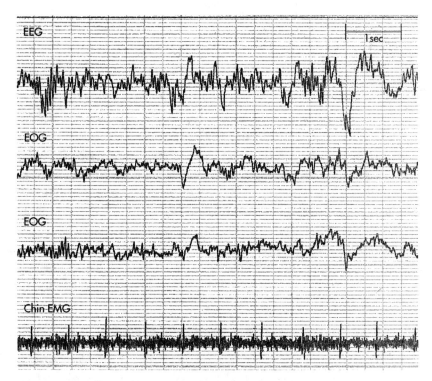

Fig. 2-2 A typical sleep recording. *EEG*, electroencephalograph or brain waves; *EOG*, electrooculograph or eye movements; *EMG*, electromyograph or muscle tension.

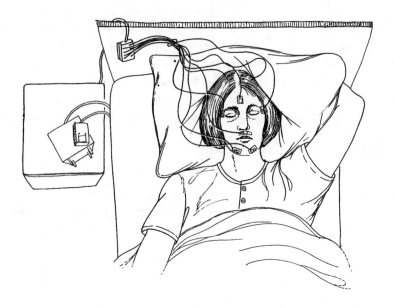

change the most during the different types of sleep. To study sleep disorders, we might also record heart rate, breathing, limb movements, the amount of oxygen in the blood, and other physiologic variables. Each variable is recorded on a polygraph, a machine that displays the biologic information as squiggly lines on a graph (Fig. 2-2). The recording of these variables is called polysomnography, from the Greek roots *poly* (many), *somno* (sleep), and *graphy* (graph). You might wonder how anyone could possibly sleep attached to all the wires required for testing. For patients whose main complaint is excessive sleepiness, sleeping attached to wires is no problem. The sleep of those complaining of insomnia may be slightly disturbed, but if a sleep disorder is present, the sleep doctor can still make a diagnosis.

WHAT ARE THE DIFFERENT TYPES OF SLEEP?

Normal sleep is made up of two distinct states. Each state is characterized by the amplitude and frequency of brain waves and the presence or absence of eye movements and muscle tension. When we are awake, our brains produce brain waves called beta waves, which primarily are in the frequency greater than 12 cycles per second. When we are relaxed but awake, our brains produce alpha waves in the frequency of 8 to 13 cycles per second. As we get sleepier, the brain waves progress to theta (4 to 7 cycles per second) and delta waves (less than 4 cycles per second).

The first state of sleep is called non–rapid eye movement sleep (NREM sleep). Non–rapid eye movement sleep is subdivided into four stages. Stage 1 is the very lightest level of sleep, the period when you are just dozing off and are not completely asleep yet, but not fully awake anymore either. Stage 1 sleep is the level of sleep in which we may find ourselves when we doze off in a dark lecture hall or at the symphony. Stage 1 sleep is characterized by some alpha activity but primarily consists of theta brain waves. There also is high activity in the chin muscle, and there may be some slow rolling eye movements. Stage 2 sleep often is considered the official onset of sleep. The EEG is characterized by sleep spindles (brief periods of activity in the 12 to 14 cycles per second range) with low muscle tension. Stages 3 and 4 get progressively deeper, with stage 4 being the very deepest level of sleep. In fact, stages 3 and 4 sometimes are lumped together and are called deep sleep or slow wave sleep (slow wave because the frequency of the brain waves is slow). Both stages 3 and 4 are characterized by EEG delta brain waves. In stage 3 sleep 20% to 50% of the time is spent in delta waves. In stage 4 sleep greater than 50% of the time is spent in delta activity.

As mentioned in the previous material and as seen in Fig. 2-3, our eyes begin slow, rolling movements as we begin to fall asleep. This is a sign of stage 1 sleep. During the rest of NREM sleep the eyes move only very slowly. In addition, the muscle tension (which traditionally is recorded under the chin) remains at a steady level.

If you are awakened during one of these four stages of sleep, you may report some mentation or thought processes but you will not report much dreaming. Our dreaming takes place in our second state of sleep, called rapid eye movement sleep, or REM sleep. Almost all of our dreams take place in REM sleep. In REM our brains produce beta activity (similar to the awake state), but we truly are

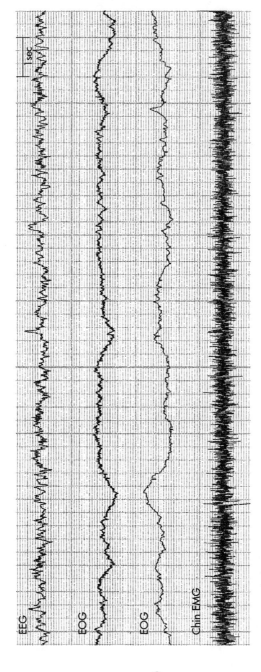

Fig. 2-3 Stage 1 sleep with slow rolling eye movements. *EEG*, electroencephalograph or brain waves; *EOG*, electrooculograph or eye movements; *EMG*, electromyograph or muscle tension.

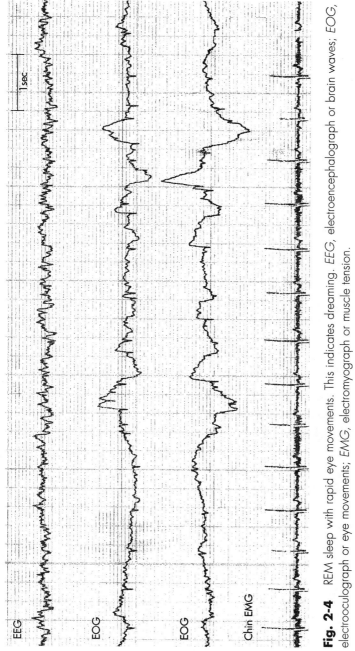

Fig. 2-4 REM sleep with rapid eye movements. This indicates dreaming. *EEG*, electroencephalograph or brain waves; *EOG*, electrooculograph or eye movements; *EMG*, electromyograph or muscle tension.

asleep. Rapid eye movement sleep sometimes is called paradoxical sleep, since the brain waves are similar to those seen during wake, for example, beta waves. As shown in Fig. 2-4, the eyes move very rapidly in bursts, thus the name "rapid eye movement sleep." In addition, notice that muscle tension is essentially flat or absent. In fact, during REM sleep, we are paralyzed except for our eyes and our respiration. This is believed to be a protective mechanism that keeps us from acting out our dreams. For example, if you are dreaming that you are jogging or playing tennis, this paralysis keeps you from jogging or practicing your backhand while in bed. Everyone dreams, but not everyone remembers his or her dreams. We are most likely to remember our dreams if we wake up during or immediately after the dream. If we stay asleep, the memory of the dream is lost.

HOW MUCH TIME DO WE SPEND IN EACH STAGE?

About 75% of the night is spent in NREM sleep. This is distributed as 5% in stage 1, 45% in stage 2, 12% in stage 3, and 13% in stage 4. Another 25% of the night is spent in REM sleep. However, we do not stay in each stage continuously, but cycle in and out of the five stages of sleep (Fig. 2-5). This cycling is called our sleep architecture. In fact, REM and NREM sleep alternate with each other throughout the night in cycles of about 80 to 100 minutes. The amount of time spent in each stage of sleep and the cycles of sleep do change as we get older.

Sleep begins with stage 1 sleep (a) and progresses through stage 2 (b) to stages 3 and 4 (c). Stage 2 (d) returns before we go on into our first REM period (e). Our first REM period occurs generally 90 to 100 minutes after we go to sleep. We then continue to cycle in and out of all the stages of sleep.

As shown in Figure 2-5, most of our deep sleep occurs in the first third of the night and most of our REM sleep occurs in the last third of the night, in the early morning hours. This tendency continues during the day as well. For example, if you take a late afternoon nap, you are more likely to go into deep sleep. If you take an early morn-

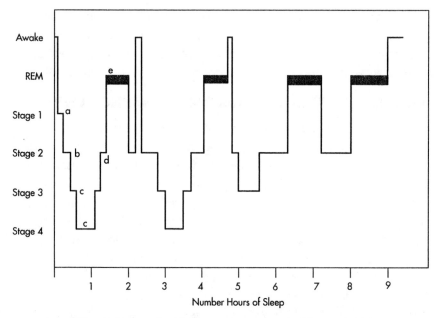

Fig. 2-5   Cycles of sleep in a young or middle-aged adult.

ing nap, you are more likely to go into REM (dream) sleep. Since REM sleep takes place in the morning, you often wake up out of REM sleep and therefore might experience "sleep paralysis"—feeling as though you cannot move or feeling very heavy when you first wake up. This is a normal feeling to experience on waking up. It would not be normal to experience this sleep paralysis on falling asleep (see Chapter 6).

DO THESE CYCLES CHANGE WITH AGE?

Infants spend almost 50% of each 24-hour day in REM sleep. In fact, newborns spend almost all their time in either active (REM) sleep or quiet (NREM) sleep. At about 6 months of age the different levels of NREM sleep begin to develop. At about the same time, the infant begins to develop more established sleep/wake cycles, beginning to sleep through the night and sleeping less during the day.

At about 20 years of age the amount of NREM sleep begins to diminish gradually. As we continue to age, the sleep cycle continues to change. In general, older people have less deep sleep and less REM sleep. These changes are described in detail in Chapter 11.

WHAT ELSE HAPPENS TO OUR BODIES DURING SLEEP?

Other physiologic systems in our bodies are also active during sleep. Our heart rates and our breathing slow down and become very regular during NREM periods as compared with wakefulness. Muscle tension decreases but stays at a steady state. But during REM sleep these systems (heart rate, respiration, blood pressure) become very irregular, speeding up and slowing down almost at random. During REM sleep we also lose control of body temperature regulation, so we are more likely to get cold if the room is cold or get hot if the room is hot.

Men experience penile erections during REM sleep. The erections have nothing to do with dreaming or with sexual desire, but rather are part of the physiologic process of REM sleep. There is also a female counterpart with women experiencing vaginal and clitoral swelling during REM sleep.

Rapid eye movement sleep behaviors are divided into two types. The first is called tonic, meaning that these behaviors occur throughout the REM period. Tonic behaviors include the suppressed EMG, elevated brain temperature, and penile erections. The second type of activity is called phasic, meaning that the behaviors occur periodically throughout the REM period. These include the rapid eye movements, tongue movements, some muscle or limb twitches, and variable heart rate and blood pressure.

The endocrine system remains active during sleep. Growth hormone, prolactin, melatonin, and thyroid hormone are secreted during deep sleep (Fig. 2-6). In fact, growth hormone is tied directly to deep sleep. If the timing of deep sleep changes, growth hormone secretion occurs during the new time of deep sleep. Steroids are secreted during REM sleep. The body temperature also cycles, with the lowest point in the early morning hours and the highest point in the late afternoon (see Chapter 8).

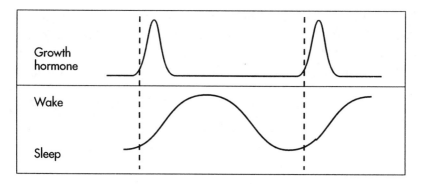

Fig. 2-6 Growth hormone cycle and sleep cycle.

HOW MUCH SLEEP DO WE NEED?

Most research has shown that the average individual needs 8 to 9 hours of sleep. This has been determined by testing hundreds of individuals with daytime performance tests after they slept different amounts of time. Most people perform best after 8 to 9 hours of sleep. But as with anything, there are individual differences. Few people need only 4 to 5 hours of sleep, while others might need 10 or more hours of sleep. Each individual can determine the amount he needs by figuring out how many hours of sleep allow him to function at an optimal level during the day. Functioning at an optimal level means not falling asleep in a dark lecture hall or while watching television or reading, but managing to stay awake no matter how boring or how quiet or how dark the environment is.

WHEN IS SLEEP ABNORMAL?

Sleep is something that happens automatically for most people. Sleep becomes abnormal when it takes you too long to fall asleep, when you wake up too often during the night and then have difficulty falling back to sleep, when your sleep is disturbed by things happening in your body or by things happening in the environment around you, when you wake up feeling tired and unrefreshed, or when you fall asleep during the day at inappropriate times. In general, sleep problems can be broken down into two categories—problems that make it difficult to sleep at night and problems that make it difficult to stay awake during the day. We will now review all the major sleep disorders, including what causes them and what can be done to improve them.

3) INSOMNIA
Why Can't I Sleep?

WHAT IS INSOMNIA?

Insomnia is not a sleep disorder! Rather, insomnia is a *complaint* of difficulty falling asleep, difficulty staying asleep, or unrestorative sleep. The complaint of insomnia can be caused by multiple factors.

The duration of the insomnia complaint is often an important clue to determining the underlying cause of the problem. Transient

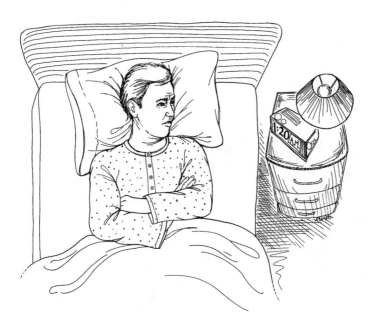

insomnia lasts only a few days and usually occurs in people who are otherwise healthy but are undergoing sudden stress (including positive stress such as getting ready for a wedding or a trip) or experiencing the onset of a medical or psychiatric illness, changes in medications, or jet lag. An example of transient insomnia would be trouble sleeping before an important exam or an important meeting.

Transient insomnia rarely is discussed in the doctor's office since it usually gets better before the patient can get an appointment. Patients usually seek professional help after experiencing short-term insomnia, which can last up to 3 weeks, or chronic insomnia, which lasts more than 3 weeks.

Chronic insomnia often is a multi-level problem, reflecting multiple predisposing, precipitating, and perpetuating factors. For example, insomnia in an already anxious individual (predisposing factor) may result from nervousness about a new job (precipitating factor). This may lead to inappropriate use of alcohol and sleeping pills at night to induce sleep, as well as increased anxiety about sleep (perpetuating factors).

WHAT CAUSES INSOMNIA?

Insomnia usually is caused by either behavioral problems and bad sleep habits, medical problems, psychiatric problems, medications and drugs, circadian rhythm disorders, or sleep disorders (such as sleep disordered breathing or periodic limb movements in sleep).

Causes of Insomnia

- Behavioral
- Medical
- Psychiatric
- Drugs
- Circadian rhythm disturbances
- Sleep disorders

Borrowed with permission from the National Sleep Foundation.

WHAT ARE BEHAVIORAL PROBLEMS THAT CAUSE INSOMNIA?

No matter what originally caused the complaint of insomnia, behavioral problems often are the main perpetuating problem. The two more common behavioral conditions are psychophysiologic insomnia and poor sleep hygiene.

Psychophysiologic insomnia occurs when you are negatively conditioned to sleeping in your bed. For example, you experience some anxiety over an upcoming job evaluation. You go to bed and have difficulty falling asleep. The next night you tell yourself that you didn't sleep well the night before, so you *have to* get some sleep tonight. You become so tense trying to sleep that you have difficulty sleeping the second night. On the third night the same thing happens. By the fourth night, even though your performance evaluation has been completed (and you received a very positive evaluation), you are very tense when you go to bed; because you now know that when you go to bed you will not be able to sleep. The transient insomnia has developed into a learned response, that is, "I won't be able to sleep when I get into bed." In fact, these patients have no trouble sleeping in the sleep laboratory or on the sofa in the living room—their main anxiety arises when they have to sleep in their own bed. Patients with psychophysiologic insomnia experience anxiety about going to sleep at night, are tired in the day because they do not sleep well, and often nap during the day.

Poor sleep hygiene means bad sleep habits. Bad sleep habits generally result from irregular sleep schedules, excessive daytime napping, overuse of alcohol and caffeine, poor sleep environments, or anxiety at bedtime. Both psychophysiologic insomnia and poor sleep hygiene can be treated by teaching the patient appropriate sleep hygiene rules. In fact, good sleep hygiene is the cornerstone of all insomnia treatments.

WHAT ARE THE RULES OF GOOD SLEEP HYGIENE?

1. *Curtail time in bed.* The longer you stay in bed, the more fragmented your sleep becomes. The less time you stay in bed, the

17

more consolidated your sleep. Therefore 8 hours of sleep out of 8.5 hours in bed is more efficient than 8 hours of sleep out of 10 hours in bed.

2. *Get up at the same time each day.* Our bodies are controlled by circadian rhythms. The circadian rhythm needs one stable point around which it can stabilize. Since you cannot control what time you fall asleep, the only time you can control is what time you wake up. Therefore it is extremely important for insomniacs to get up at the same time each day (including weekends) and to avoid "sleeping in."

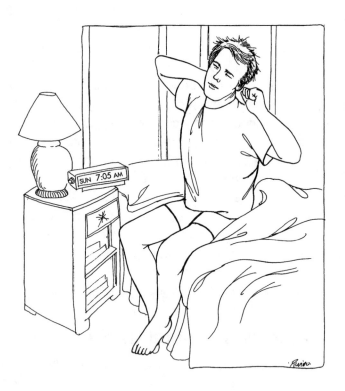

3. *Avoid the bedroom clock.* The first thing you do when you wake up in the middle of the night is look at your clock. The time pressure contributes to poor sleep. In addition, the acts of opening your eyes to see the clock and lifting your head to read the time wake you up even more. What difference does it make if it is 1:00 AM or 3:00 AM? Turn your clock around or move it to the other side of the room where you won't be tempted to look. If you wake up in the middle of the night, keep your eyes closed, and you will be more likely to go right back to sleep.

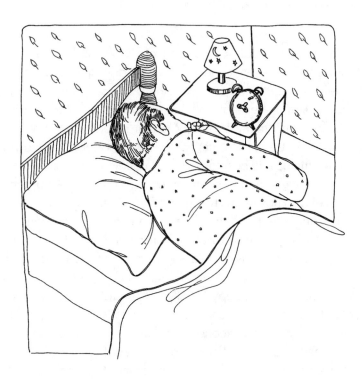

Amount of Caffeine in Chocolate and in Sodas:

Chocolate*	Caffeine (milligrams)	12 oz Soda†	Caffeine (milligrams)
1.5 oz. Dark chocolate	31	Mountain Dew	54
1.5 oz Milk chocolate	9	Coca-Cola	46
5 oz Hot chocolate	8	Dr. Pepper	41
5 oz Chocolate milk	1.25	Pepsi Cola/Diet Pepsi	35
1 Hershey's Kiss	1.2	7-Up/Diet 7-Up	0
2 tablespoons Chocolate fudge	5	Sprite	0
1/4 cup Semisweet		Hires Root Beer	0
chocolate chips	33	Diet Sunkist Orange	0

*Modified from Aytur S: Chocolate. In Carskadon M, editor: *Encyclopedia of sleep and dreaming*, New York, 1993, Macmillan.
†Modified from Coffee and health, *Consumer Reports*, p 651, Oct 1994.

4. *Avoid caffeine, alcohol, and tobacco.* Caffeine has been shown to disrupt sleep, even in individuals who don't think it affects them. The effect of caffeine remains in the body on average from 3 to 5 hours. Remember that caffeine is not just in coffee but in tea, chocolate, and many sodas (note that a soda does not have to be brown to be full of caffeine—read the labels). For individuals with insomnia, it is best to avoid all caffeine after lunchtime.

And if you need one more reason to stop smoking, tobacco (nicotine) also has been shown to disturb sleep. Nicotine can have an arousing effect and therefore make it more difficult to sleep.

Alcohol often is used by insomniacs to help them fall asleep. One old wives' tale suggests having a glass of sherry before bed to promote sleep. In fact this is just an old wives' tale. Alcohol makes you sleepy initially but several hours later when the alcohol wears off, it can cause you to wake up (insomnia). Therefore if you drink alcohol with dinner, you may be sleepy right after dinner, but several hours later, when it is time for bed, you may be wide awake. If you drink alcohol right before bedtime,

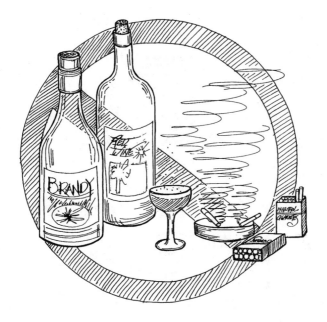

you may fall asleep quicker but several hours later, at 1:00 or 2:00 in the morning, you may wake up again and have difficulty going back to sleep.

5. *Exercise.* Keeping generally fit will promote sleep. Exercising right before bedtime may make sleep more difficult, because one of our circadian rhythms is the body temperature cycle. When our body temperature drops, we become sleepy. Exercising increases our body temperature. It then takes about 6 hours for the body temperature to begin to drop; at that point it will be easier to fall asleep. Therefore exercising about 6 hours before bedtime promotes sleep.

6. *Eat a light snack.* Going to bed with an empty, hungry stomach makes it more difficult to sleep. Eating a light snack, particularly one with tryptophan, helps promote sleep. Tryptophan is a naturally produced amino acid with sleep-promoting properties and can be found in products such as milk, cheese, bananas, fish,

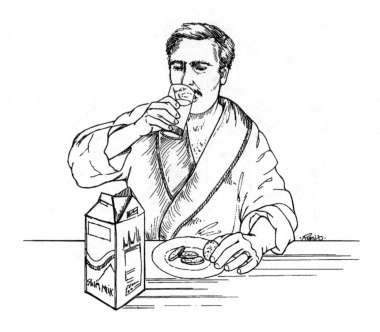

and turkey. (Why do you think you are so tired after your Thanksgiving meal?). Therefore a glass of warm milk at bedtime may be quite conducive to sleep.

7. *Adjust sleeping environment.* The sleep environment should be relaxing, comfortable, and conducive to sleep. If the bedroom is too noisy, consider moving to a quieter room in the house or using ear plugs. If there is too much light, try dark curtains or eye shades.

8. *Do not worry right before bed.* Generally in our busy schedules, the first time we have to sit quietly and think about our day is when we get into bed. This is the wrong time to start worrying. Plan a quiet time earlier in the evening that will allow you time to think, plan, and "worry" away from your bedroom, thus interfering less with sleep. If you find it helpful to write things down, this is the time to make lists of all the different options you have for the things you are worrying about.

In summary, sleep hygiene rules are:

1. Curtail time in bed.
2. Get up at the same time each day.
3. Avoid bedroom clock.
4. Avoid caffeine, alcohol, and tobacco.
5. Exercise.
6. Eat a light snack.
7. Adjust sleeping environment.
8. Do not worry right before bed.

ARE THERE BEHAVIORAL TREATMENTS FOR INSOMNIA?

Behavioral treatments, in combination with sleep hygiene, may be helpful in treating psychophysiologic and other insomnias. Relaxation training (such as progressive relaxation, biofeedback, meditation, deep breathing, or counting sheep) can be effective if practiced until relaxation becomes automatic.

Progressive relaxation training is effective if your tension is physical, for example, if you have difficulty relaxing your muscles. Lie down on your back in bed with the lights out. Close your eyes, and breathe deeply several times. Continue to breathe deeply throughout the exercise. Begin with your toes. While leaving the rest of your body relaxed, tense your toes by curling them down. Notice how tight they feel. Then relax. Continue tightening and relaxing each muscle group working up the body: toes, calves, thighs, stomach, shoulders, hands, arms, neck, face. With each tightening keep breathing and pay attention to what the muscles feel like when they are tense compared with what they feel like when you relax them. Tightening the muscles acts as a pendulum, allowing you to relax more deeply than if you didn't tense first. This exercise can be practiced during the day as well. The more often you practice the exercise, the more relaxed you will become, and the more effective the exercise will be.

23

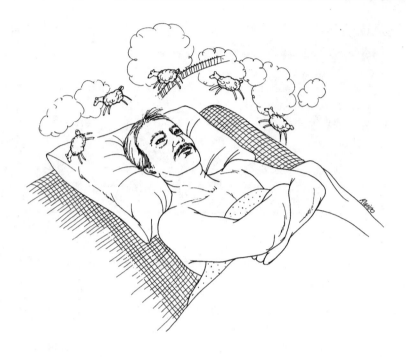

Breathing deeply and counting your breaths (or sheep) helps relax an active mind. Take a deep breath and count one. Focus on the breathing. Take a second deep breath and count two. If your mind wanders (and it will), go back to counting from one. With practice you will be able to count to ten and be asleep before you know it.

Two other behavioral therapies have been shown to be effective for insomnia. They are stimulus-control therapy, developed by Dr. Richard Bootzin, and sleep restriction therapy, developed by Dr. Arthur Spielman. These techniques are best when done under the supervision of a behavioral therapist or sleep specialist. They are described here for informational purposes.

Stimulus-Control Therapy

The aim of stimulus-control therapy is to break the negative associations of being in bed but unable to sleep. It is especially helpful for

24

patients with sleep-onset insomnia and prolonged midsleep awakenings. The rules of stimulus-control therapy include:

1. Only go to bed when you feel sleepy.
2. If you don't fall asleep within 15 minutes, get out of bed and
   don't go back to bed until you think you can fall asleep. If you
   go back to bed and still can't fall asleep, get out of bed again.
   Repeat this until you can fall asleep within a few minutes.
3. Avoid looking at the clock.
4. Get up at the same time every morning.
5. Use the bed only for sleeping, not for watching the evening
   news, paying bills, reading exciting books, etc.
6. Do not nap during the day.

After the first night you will be very sleepy and should be extra
careful if you have to drive or use special equipment during the day.
The second night you should have an easier time falling asleep. If
not, repeat the instructions listed previously. In all it may take 3 to 4
weeks, but after breaking the unwanted pattern, you should have little difficulty falling asleep at night.

Sleep Restriction Therapy

Sleep restriction therapy is based on the observation that the more
time spent in bed leads to more fragmented sleep, and conversely,
the less time spent in bed, the more consolidated sleep becomes. The
rules of sleep restriction therapy include:

1. You only are allowed to stay in bed for the amount of time
   you think you sleep each night, plus 15 minutes. For example, if you report sleeping only 5 hours a night, you are
   allowed to be in bed for 5 hours and 15 minutes.
2. You must get up at the same time each day. If you sleep for
   5 hours and generally get up at 6:00 AM, you are allowed
   to be in bed from 12:45 AM until 6:00 AM.

3. Do not nap during the day.
4. When you are asleep for 85% of the time you stay in bed, you can increase the amount of time in bed by going to bed 15 minutes earlier. (You still have to get up at the same time in the morning.)
5. Repeat this process until you are sleeping for 8 hours or the desired amount of time.

This procedure also takes 3 to 4 weeks to be effective. Be aware that, as with stimulus-control therapy, you may be very sleepy during the day and should be extremely careful driving, etc.

ARE THERE OTHER TYPES OF NONDRUG TREATMENTS OF INSOMNIA?

Another approach to treating insomnia, often done in combination with behavioral therapy, is called cognitive behavioral therapy (CBT). Insomnia may be exacerbated by what people believe. For example, if you think you will get sick if you don't sleep 8 hours each night, this belief can cause you to worry if on some nights you get less than 8 hours sleep. This anxiety can make insomnia worse. Or if you think that any change you experience in your sleep means something is wrong, this too can cause insomnia. Another example might be the belief that because your wife falls asleep immediately, there must be something wrong with you because it takes you longer to fall asleep. So what we believe and what we think can be a part of our sleep problem. Insomniacs often have unrealistic sleep expectations, don't understand the cause of their sleep problem, and engage in catastrophic thinking about the effect of their sleep problem.

Cognitive behavioral therapy, a type of therapy explored in detail by Charles Morin and his colleagues, consists of a combination of the behavioral therapies described in the previous material (such as sleep restriction or stimulus-control therapy) in addition to providing the individuals with alternative beliefs and changing their attitudes about sleep and about the effect lack of sleep has on daytime behavior.

Cognitive behavioral therapy involves three steps: (1) to identify the dysfunctional beliefs ("I must sleep 8 hours or I will get sick"); (2) to challenge those beliefs ("Have you ever gotten sick because you only slept 6.5 hours?" or "What is the evidence that you will get sick?"); and (3) to teach new beliefs that are more realistic ("If I don't get enough sleep tonight or tomorrow night, I may be fatigued during the day, but I won't get sick and my body will eventually take the sleep it needs."). The cognitive restructuring is aimed at decreasing the difference between the patient's reality and her beliefs about sleep. The main focus is to break the vicious cycle of worrying about loss of sleep, fear of sleeplessness, anxiety over not sleeping, and more insomnia.

WHAT TYPE OF MEDICAL PROBLEMS CAUSE INSOMNIA?

Insomnia can result from any medical problem that causes pain or discomfort. This could include illnesses such as heart disease, pulmonary disease, cancer, or arthritis. It is important to determine if the insomnia complaint is related to the medical problem by examining the time course of each. For example, if the complaint of poor sleep is worse when the pain of arthritis flares up, then it is likely that the insomnia is secondary to the pain. The first line of therapy in this type of situation is treating the medical problem and any bad sleep habits that have developed.

Patients with rheumatologic disease, which causes pain during the night, usually have no difficulty falling asleep but may experience more awakenings during the night, less overall time asleep, and more time spent in stage 1 (light) sleep. Patients taking benzodiazepines (a type of sleeping pill) have reported sleeping better and experiencing less pain at night, but their complaints of morning stiffness increase. The use of aspirin in combination with a sedative-hypnotic alleviates the morning stiffness. Tricyclic antidepressants (such as amitriptyline) also have been used successfully to treat this disorder.

Other examples of medical illnesses that are known to disturb sleep include:

- osteoarthritis, which limits movement during the night

27

- fibromyalgia, which results in chronic fatigue
- pulmonary disease (such as chronic obstructive lung disease, asthma, and chronic cough), which causes disturbed sleep secondary to difficulty breathing
- congestive heart failure, which can cause multiple awakenings during the night
- gastrointestinal problems, which lead to reflux and pain of ulcers

WHAT TYPE OF PSYCHIATRIC PROBLEMS CAUSE INSOMNIA?

Almost all patients with psychiatric disease complain of insomnia. The severity of the insomnia generally varies with the severity of the psychiatric problem. For example, early morning awakenings are associated with depression, and trouble falling asleep is associated with generalized anxiety. As with the medical conditions, treatment includes treating the primary psychiatric problem in combination with any bad sleep habits that have developed.

Depression is one of the most common causes of insomnia. Patients with depression experience fragmented sleep, difficulty falling asleep, and frequent awakenings during the night. They have decreased amounts of stage 3 and 4 (deep) sleep, decreased time to the first REM period, and increased REM sleep activity.

HOW CAN DRUGS CAUSE INSOMNIA?

Many medications have an effect on sleep. Many drugs are stimulating and if taken in the evening, cause insomnia. Other drugs are depressants and if taken in the day, cause daytime sleepiness. Sleeping pills, with long-term use, may even cause insomnia. If you are taking sleeping pills and suddenly decide to stop, you will experience rebound insomnia. This means that for the first night or so, your insomnia actually gets worse. A natural reaction is to think, "Oh, I can't sleep without my sleeping pill," and you go back to taking the drugs. In fact, it takes some time for your body to adjust to the rebound insomnia, and if you are patient and give yourself a few nights of bad sleep, you actually may begin to sleep better. Drugs are discussed more fully in Chapter 12.

HOW COMMON IS INSOMNIA?

In data collected by the Gallup Poll for the National Sleep Foundation, 9% of the population reported chronic insomnia and 27% reported transient or intermittent insomnia during the course of a year. The complaint of insomnia is more common in women than men, increases with age, and is more common in lower socioeconomic classes. The most common problem reported was waking up feeling drowsy. Chronic insomniacs reported more difficulty enjoying family and social relationships, more difficulty concentrating, more problems with memory, greater frequency of falling asleep while visiting friends, and more automobile accidents resulting from sleepiness. Younger insomniacs generally have a complaint of difficulty falling asleep, whereas older insomniacs generally have a complaint of staying asleep.

WHEN SHOULD I SEE MY DOCTOR?

It is time to see your doctor when your insomnia is routinely disrupting your everyday life. Remember, insomnia is a real complaint caused by real problems. And also remember, there is help for insomnia.

4) HYPERSOMNIA
Why Do I Sleep So Much?

Hypersomnia means sleeping too much or being overly sleepy. People with hypersomnia usually are excessively sleepy during the day. This symptom is called excessive daytime sleepiness or EDS.

WHAT CAUSES HYPERSOMNIA?

Hypersomnia generally is caused by lack of sleep during the night. The body needs a certain amount of sleep every 24 hours. For most people, that means about 8 hours of sleep. When that sleep is not obtained at night, your body tries to catch up on the sleep during the day. The bigger question becomes, why is your body not getting enough sleep at night? Are you sleep deprived because you are going to bed too late and getting up too early? Are you sleepy during the day because of problems with insomnia at night? Sleep may be disturbed by specific sleep disorders such as sleep-disordered breathing (see Chapter 5), periodic limb movements in sleep (see Chapter 7), or narcolepsy (see Chapter 6). Medical illness or psychiatric illness can also cause daytime sleepiness. Certain medications (such as tranquilizers) also have the side effect of causing daytime sleepiness or hypersomnia. Withdrawal from other medications (such as caffeine) also can cause sleepiness.

CAN HAVING HYPERSOMNIA BE SERIOUS?

Hypersomnia can cause difficulties with memory and concentration, thus affecting performance. This can become especially dangerous when poor performance resulting from sleepiness leads to accidents.

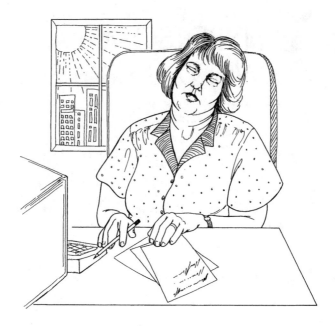

The famous Exxon Valdez accident, which occurred in 1989 and created a major oil spill in the waters of Alaska, was caused by the ship being left in charge of a third mate who not only was under-qualified, but who also was overtired from his overloaded schedule of duties. Fatigue also has been cited as the most frequent cause of fatal accidents in truck drivers. The U.S. Department of Transportation estimates that about 200,000 traffic accidents each year are most likely a result of sleep problems and that of all drivers in the United States, 20% have dozed off at least once while driving.

HOW COMMON IS HYPERSOMNIA?

It has been estimated that about 4% to 5% of the population suffers from excessive daytime sleepiness. However, the true number is difficult to determine since many people believe it is normal it be sleepy during the day (and to take regular naps) and do not report the EDS as a problem.

HOW IS HYPERSOMNIA TREATED?

The treatment of hypersomnia first involves determining what is causing the sleepiness. If the sleepiness is caused by medication, then the
physician may adjust the dose and time of day the medication is
taken. If the hypersomnia is caused by sleep deprivation (that is, not
getting enough sleep at night), the treatment may be as simple as
sleeping more hours at night. If the hypersomnia is caused by illness
(such as sleep apnea), then the physician must treat the illness. The
following four chapters explain some of the sleep disorders that have
hypersomnia, or EDS, as a major complaint.

5 ⟩ SLEEP DISORDERED BREATHING

Breathing is one of those things that you never have to think about doing. Your body just does it. Unfortunately however, sometimes during sleep, the body either forgets to breathe, has a hard time breathing, or is unable to pass air even when trying to breathe. This is called sleep disordered breathing (SDB).

Sleep disordered breathing, also called sleep apnea, was first described in the late 1800s. Yet it was only 25 years ago that doctors recognized it as a serious problem. The word *apnea* comes from the Greek words "a," which means absence of, and "pnoia," which means breath. Sleep apnea syndrome is defined as breathing that temporarily stops during sleep. You fall asleep; you stop breathing; to start breathing again, you wake up; you start breathing; you fall back to sleep; you stop breathing. This cycle continues throughout the night. The awakenings you experience are so brief that you are not aware of them, but they are long enough to help you start breathing again and long enough to disrupt your sleep.

For the diagnosis of SDB to be made, each apnea episode must last a minimum of 10 seconds and must occur at least 5 times for each hour you are asleep. This is called the apnea index (AI; number of apneas per hour of sleep). Partial decreases in breathing, called hypopneas, may also produce brief awakenings even when complete apneas do not occur. Therefore, rather than using just the apnea index, a respiratory disturbance index (RDI; number of respiratory events, or number of apneas plus hypopneas per hour of sleep) is used. Although the criterion for RDI has not been fully established, many clinicians use 10 to 15 events per hour of sleep for the purpose of diagnosis.

Clinically, it is not unusual to see patients being evaluated for sleep apnea who have a much higher number of apneas and hypopneas than the minimum required for diagnosis—for example, they may stop breathing for 60 to 120 seconds with each event, and experience hundreds of events per night. Many individuals with SDB cannot sleep and breathe at the same time and therefore spend most of the night not sleeping and not breathing.

WHAT CAUSES SLEEP DISORDERED BREATHING?

The most common type of SDB is obstructive sleep apnea. Normally, the air you breathe passes from your nose and mouth through your throat to your lungs. The portion of the throat just above the larynx (the voice box) is soft and flexible so you can swallow and so you can make the sounds needed for whispering, talking, singing, and yelling.

The soft palate is the tissue at the back of the roof of your mouth that blocks the passage leading to your nose when you swallow. This prevents food from going up into your nose. The uvula is the flap that hangs down in the back of your throat. Your tonsils are globules of tissue far back on both sides of the throat that frequently swell and become tender during throat infections, especially in children. Muscles hold the airway open by keeping each structure tight and in place. During sleep the muscles relax some, but in a normal individual, air can still pass. When any of these structures is anatomically abnormal, air is prevented from freely flowing during sleep, causing snoring and SDB.

Obstructive sleep apnea occurs when the muscles of the airway collapse, resulting in partial or complete blockage of airflow. You still attempt to breathe, your diaphragm is still moving, but the collapse of the airway muscles blocks your airway, so the air cannot get in or out. Therefore the reason you stop breathing is that when you fall asleep, the muscles in your airway collapse, blocking the air from going through. When you wake up, even briefly, the airway opens again. This is similar to what would happen with paper straws. Before straws were made of plastic, they were made of paper. When you sucked very hard on a wet paper straw, the walls of the straw would collapse. This is exactly what happens in your airway.

36

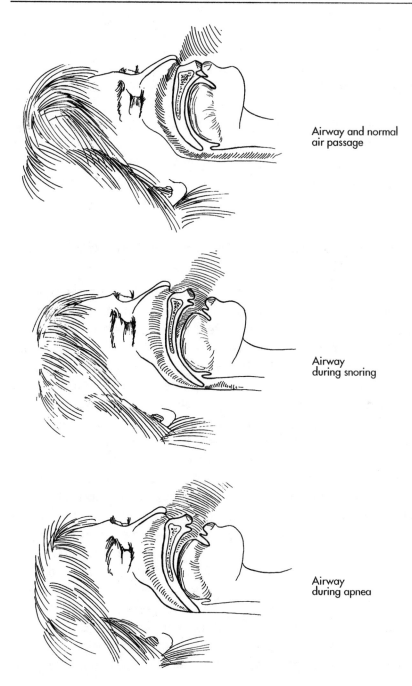

Airway and normal
air passage

Airway
during snoring

Airway
during apnea

The airway collapse of obstructive sleep apnea can be caused by bagginess or excessive pharyngeal tissue, a large uvula, fatty deposits at the base of the tongue, or collapse of the pharyngeal walls. The resulting decreased air passage compromises ventilation, thus causing the amount of oxygen in the blood to drop.

Since air also flows through the nose, blockage of the nasal passages also can cause problems and potentially make sleep apnea worse. A deviated septum (the wall between your two nostrils is crooked and blocks one side of your nose); enlarged tonsils; or blockage resulting from allergies, colds, or polyps (growths), can all make SDB, and snoring, worse.

ARE THERE OTHER TYPES OF SLEEP DISORDERED BREATHING?

Other types of sleep disordered breathing exist. Central sleep apnea results from failure of the respiratory centers in the brain to stimulate the motor neurons that control breathing. No attempt to breathe is made, and although the airway is not collapsed, no respiration occurs. This type of apnea is less common and usually is associated with heart disease or neurologic disease, although sometimes we cannot identify a cause.

Mixed sleep apnea, as the name implies, is a combination of obstructive and central sleep apnea. It usually begins with a central component, that is, there is no breathing. Suddenly the diaphragm begins to move, but the airway is still blocked, that is, the obstructive component. It is not uncommon to see patients have obstructive, central, and mixed sleep apneas occur all on the same night.

Periodic breathing is breathing in which the amount of respiration increases and decreases in a cyclic pattern (described as a crescendo and decrescendo pattern by musicians). It can occur while awake, but is frequently more noticeable and more severe during sleep. It is often associated with heart disease but can occur in normal subjects during the first few days at high altitudes.

Hypoventilation is breathing that is somewhat below normal in volume. Small decreases in breathing during sleep are common and normal. In some patients with lung disease or in those with marked obesity, the normal small decreases in breathing that occur with sleep can result in decreases in blood oxygen levels and, in severe cases, this can lead to heart problems.

WHAT ARE THE SYMPTOMS OF SLEEP DISORDERED BREATHING?

The most common symptoms of SDB that bring the patient in to see the doctor are excessive daytime sleepiness and snoring. The excessive daytime sleepiness is believed to be caused by the frequent awakenings occurring at the end of the apneas. The drop in oxygen also may contribute to the excessive sleepiness. When breathing becomes more difficult or actually stops during sleep, alarms go off in your brain that cause you to awaken or partially awaken by moving from deeper stages of sleep to lighter stages of sleep. Once you partially awaken, breathing is restored to its normal awake levels. Soon after breathing is restored and you fall back to sleep, the breathing problems begin again to be followed by another awakening. Such cycles can continue for many minutes, hours, or throughout the night, resulting in significant decreases in the amount of time spent sleeping. So, the next day, you are still very tired.

Patients with excessive daytime sleepiness fall asleep at inappropriate times—basically, whenever they are sitting quietly. Complaints may vary from mild lethargy and decreased concentration to more extreme complaints such as falling asleep at your desk at work, while reading or writing or watching television, while sitting in conversation with a group of people, while at a meeting, or while driving. A distinction must be made between excessive daytime sleepiness and naps taken on purpose. ("I'm tired so I think I'll lie down and take a nap.") These inadvertent naps of excessive sleepiness are more of an uncontrollable urge to close your eyes and fall asleep. Most often, you will not realize you have fallen asleep until you suddenly wake up or are awakened.

The second very common complaint is loud snoring. The bed partner usually has complained about the loud snoring for years and

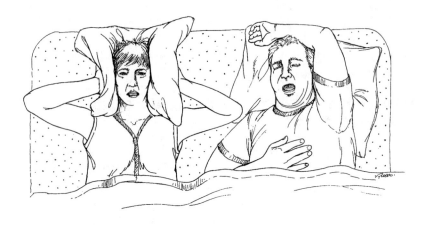

either has threatened to move out of the bedroom or has already moved out. The snoring often is loud enough to be heard throughout the house. Bed partners describe a characteristic pattern of loud snoring interrupted by periods of silence that are then terminated by snorting sounds.

Snoring results from a partial narrowing of the airway caused by multiple factors such as inadequate muscle tone, large tonsils and adenoids, long soft palate, and/or limp tissue. Snoring has been implicated not only in sleep apnea, but also in stroke and heart disease, even without complete sleep apneas. The prevalence of snoring increases with age, especially in women. It is important to note that snoring is not always a symptom of SDB. Approximately 25% of men and 15% of women are habitual snorers.

Patients with SDB frequently are overweight. In some patients, a weight gain of 20 to 30 pounds might bring on episodes of sleep disordered breathing. The same fatty tissue seen on the outside is also present on the inside, making the airway even more narrow. The more you weigh, the worse the symptoms of SDB will be. Since obstructive sleep apnea always is caused by the collapse of the airway, in patients of normal weight, anatomic abnormalities (such as large tonsils, long uvula, etc.) must be considered.

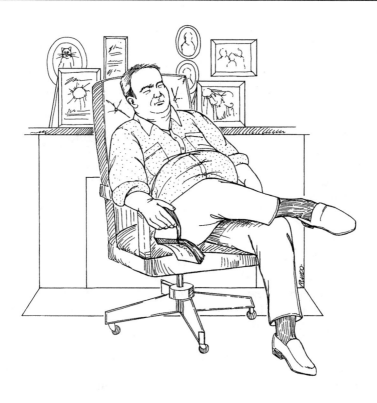

Sleep disordered breathing is also associated with heart disease, hypertension, morning headaches, dry mouth on awakening, excessive movements during the night, falling out of bed, bedwetting, cognitive decline and personality changes, and complaints of insomnia. The typical patient with obstructive sleep apnea is a middle-aged male who is overweight or who has an anatomically narrow upper airway.

The heart irregularities seen with sleep apnea syndrome include bradycardia (the heart slows down) during the apnea events and tachycardia (the heart speeds up) after the end of the events. It is not unusual to see other types of irregular heart rhythms. However, the heart recording taken during the waking state might be normal. It only is during the apneas and hypopneas during sleep that the abnormalities appear.

Nocturnal hypertension (that is, high blood pressure) also is very common in these patients. About 50% of patients with SDB have hypertension and about one third of all hypertensives have SDB. However, in addition to the daytime hypertension, blood pressure rises during respiratory events in sleep.

HOW DO I KNOW IF I HAVE SLEEP DISORDERED BREATHING?

There are several clues that you can look for to decide if you might have SDB and whether you should see your doctor. These signs include:

- Your bed partner mentions that she or he has noticed that you stop breathing.
- Your bed partner has moved out or has threatened to move out of the bedroom because you snore so loudly.
- Other people living in the house can hear you snore.
- You feel tired or fatigued in the morning even when you feel that you got a good, long night's sleep.
- You wake up with a headache on a regular basis.
- You are having difficulty with your memory and/or concentration.
- You find yourself falling asleep or fighting to stay awake at meetings, at church or synagogue, at work, while in conversation with friends, or at other inappropriate times.
- You have had multiple near-miss accidents because you fell asleep driving.
- You have had a car accident caused by your falling asleep.

IF I SUSPECT SLEEP APNEA, WHAT SHOULD I DO?

If you have these symptoms or you suspect you might have SDB, you should see your doctor immediately. If you are overweight, you should begin a weight loss program. In addition, you should avoid sleeping pills and alcohol.

Sleeping pills are respiratory depressants. That means they make it harder to breathe. Sleeping pills in a person with SDB will make the apneas longer, will increase the number of apneas per night, and will make it harder to wake up. (The point of the sleeping pill is to keep the individual from waking up.) However, since the person with apnea needs to wake up to start breathing again, sleeping pills can be dangerous to people with this condition.

Alcohol is also a respiratory depressant. If you suspect you have SDB, you should avoid all alcohol. In addition to making sleep disordered breathing worse, alcohol also makes snoring worse.

Other drugs might make sleep disordered breathing worse. Narcotics, such as morphine, and anesthetics are respiratory depressants. If you have SDB and are about to undergo surgery with the use of a general anesthetic, it is a good idea to talk to your surgeon and your anesthesiologist about your condition. With proper preparation, there should be no problems. However, if the doctors performing the surgery are not aware of your problem, you may be at risk for respiratory failure during the surgery.

HOW WILL MY DOCTOR DETERMINE IF I HAVE SLEEP DISORDERED BREATHING?

Your doctor will begin by asking you questions about your medical history, your medication or drug use, your sleep habits, your daytime activities, your diet, your use of alcohol, and other various questions that help determine if you might have this disorder. If you have a bed partner, the doctor may ask your bed partner to accompany you to this visit, since your bed partner often is more aware of what you do at night (after all, you are asleep at the time). You then schedule a time to sleep in the laboratory or clinic where your sleep can be recorded. Only with an objective recording can a complete diagnosis be made. A detailed description of this procedure is provided in Chapter 12.

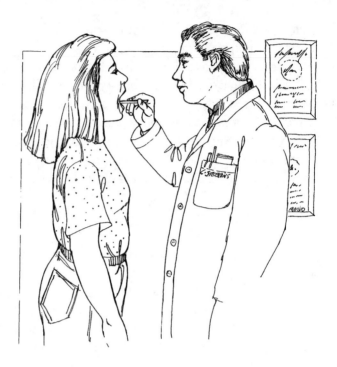

HOW COMMON IS SLEEP DISORDERED BREATHING?

Recently published research conducted by Dr. Terry Young and her colleagues, and funded by the U.S. National Institutes of Health, has demonstrated that although approximately 50% of randomly selected adults age 30 to 60 years had virtually no apneas during sleep, 4% of men and 2% of women had 5 or more apneas or hypopneas per hour of sleep. So it is not surprising if you carefully observe a friend or family member sleeping for part of the night, you may see occasional pauses in their breathing.

The prevalence of sleep apnea does increase with age. Data from my own laboratory show that the percentage of elderly with at least 5 apneas per hour of sleep is about 28% in men and 19% in women. Mild to moderate sleep-related breathing disturbances increase with age, even in elderly subjects without major complaints about their sleep. The incidence is higher in men than women, at least until the age of menopause, after which the rates in women increase and may approach those of men. In general, the severity of apnea in these older persons is mild compared with that seen in patients with clinical sleep apnea. However, older men and women with mild apnea have been reported to fall asleep at inappropriate times significantly more often than older persons without apnea. Furthermore, the incidence of sleep apnea and other sleep-related breathing disturbances is higher in individuals with hypertension, congestive heart failure, obesity, dementia, and other medical conditions.

WHAT ARE SOME CONSEQUENCES OF UNTREATED SLEEP DISORDERED BREATHING?

This is a very difficult question to answer and currently is the focus of considerable research. Several studies have now confirmed that severe sleep apnea, if left untreated, may be associated with increased risk of death, particularly in patients with heart disease or whose hearts are unable to cope with the demands of massive obesity combined with months (or years) of coping with not breathing during sleep.

The clinical significance of relatively mild sleep apneas is not yet fully understood. However, even mild SDB may be associated with either insomnia or excessive daytime sleepiness. Patients with SDB should avoid sleeping pills, alcohol, or other sedating medications since these will make it harder to breathe at night.

HOW IS SLEEP DISORDERED BREATHING TREATED?

Sleep disordered breathing and snoring hardly ever go away on their own. The good news is that they can be treated. For SDB, the preferred treatment at the time of this writing is the very inelegant but usually effective form of treatment involving an air pressure machine called continuous positive airway pressure (CPAP). A comfortable nose mask is connected by a hose to a machine that blows air. The mask is specially adapted to fit each individual's nose. The mask is worn at night, and the air blower is turned on. The air blower blows positive air pressure through the hose into your nose and airway. The positive air pressure acts almost as a splint to keep the airway open during sleep. Your doctor, or specially trained associate, will test different pressures while you sleep in the laboratory to determine which pressure is best for you. You will need to wear the CPAP mask every night. On nights that you do not use the machine, your sleep apnea will return. The CPAP does not cure the SDB, but rather helps to keep the airway open during sleep. Most machines are portable and can be taken along on vacations and business trips when you have to sleep away from home.

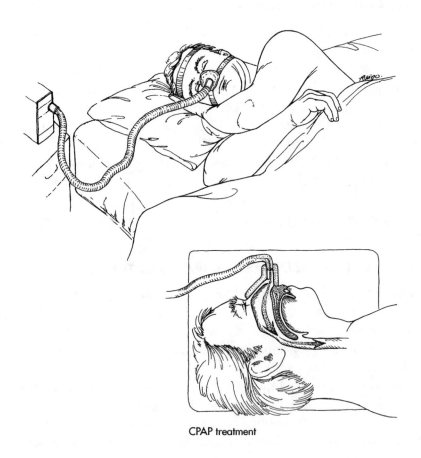

CPAP treatment

ARE THERE PROBLEMS WITH USING CONTINUOUS POSITIVE AIRWAY PRESSURE?

As with anything new, it may take a little time to adjust to the CPAP. The CPAP mask comes in many shapes and sizes. Your doctor will help you find the one that is most comfortable for you. If you decide your mask does not fit well after a few weeks, talk to your doctor about an adjustment. If your airway or nose becomes dry, a humidifier can be added to the CPAP to add some moisture to the system. If your nose is blocked due to a cold or allergies, the CPAP does not work as well; see your doctor about clearing your nasal passages.

ARE OTHER TREATMENTS AVAILABLE?

Other treatments for sleep apnea include surgery that enlarges the airway by tightening the flabby muscles in the airway, removing unnecessary tissue, and shortening the uvula. This surgery is called uvulopalatopharyngoplasty (UPPP). Although this surgery is effective for eliminating snoring, it only cures the SDB some of the time. It is extremely important for your doctor to determine if you might or might not benefit from having surgery.

The UPPP is done under general anesthesia and requires you to stay in the hospital for a few days. You will wake up with a sore throat that should go away with time. Some potential, but rare, complications of UPPP include a possible voice change and, as with any major surgery, risk of excessive bleeding or infection. Since the uvula has been shortened or removed, some people find that their food or drink flows into their nose when they swallow. This almost always resolves as you learn different ways of swallowing. However, a common consequence of the UPPP is that although the SDB may not be cured, the snoring is gone. Therefore, unless you have sleep rerecorded or are observed at night, you will not know if you still stop breathing while sleeping.

Improving the surgical therapy of sleep apnea is a focus of considerable research. Early results from surgery that opens the upper airway during sleep by pulling the tongue forward or by advancing the jaw forward, show considerable better rates of "cure" than experi-

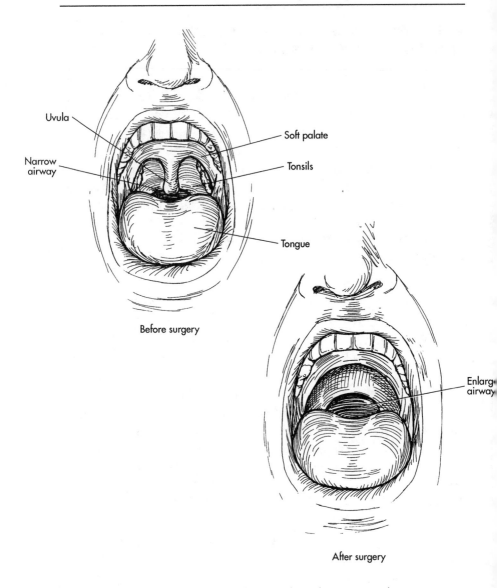

Uvula

Narrow airway

Soft palate

Tonsils

Tongue

Before surgery

Enlarge airway

After surgery

enced with UPPP alone. Consulting with a sleep specialist or surgeon experienced in such surgeries is essential for getting the most up-to-date advice as to whether surgery is an appropriate option for you and for matching the type of surgery most likely to be effective with a minimal risk of complications.

In addition to these surgical options for treating sleep apnea, there is an important new surgical procedure aimed at eliminating or reducing snoring. This surgery is called laser assisted uvula-palatoplasty (LAUP). A laser beam is used to trim the tissues at the back of the throat that otherwise vibrate while breathing during sleep. Specifically, the laser beam shortens or removes the uvula and trims the soft palate. The procedure can be done in the doctor's office with a local anesthetic. It often takes multiple visits to complete the entire procedure. After the surgery you will experience some discomfort that should improve with time. The duration of the sore throat after the LAUP surgery is much shorter than with the UPPP surgery.

The LAUP procedure is so new that there is little research or long-term follow-up data available at this time to determine the effects on sleep apnea or the long-term effectiveness on snoring. As with UPPP, the most serious complication is that people may think this surgery has cured their SDB. It may not, since the blockage that causes the SDB usually occurs farther back in the airway—much farther than the laser can reach. Other complications also can include possible voice changes, bleeding, infection, and food or drink flowing into the nose.

Mild sleep apnea is sometimes improved by weight loss. Losing as little as 20 to 30 pounds may improve the apnea in mild cases.

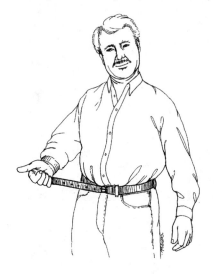

Mild sleep apnea also may be improved by changing body position during sleep. Sleeping on your back makes snoring and apneas worse. By avoiding lying on your back, you can improve both the snoring and the apneas. This is best accomplished by sewing a pocket in the back of a t-shirt or pajama top and placing a tennis ball or whiffle ball in the pocket. The ball makes it very uncomfortable to sleep on your back.

Another type of treatment is dental devices that are worn at night. Many different types of dental devices are available, and depending on the severity of your condition and the cause of your condition, your doctor can recommend the device that would be best for you. The device is fitted by a dentist who also is trained in sleep-disorders medicine. Some of the dental devices hold the tongue forward with suction to keep it from flapping back and blocking the airway. Other dental devices pull the jaw forward to enlarge the airway. As with CPAP, dental devices do not cure the sleep disordered breathing, but help to open up the airway. Therefore they too need to be used every night. Your dentist and doctor will train you on how to use your dental device and on how to care for it.

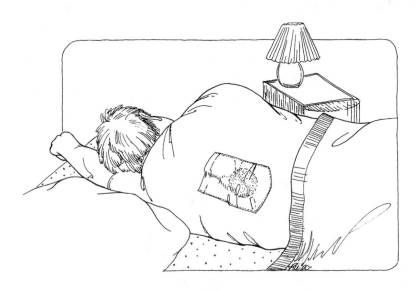

50

Sometimes SDB is treated with medications. Some of the tricyclic antidepressants, which usually are used to treat depression, also are respiratory stimulants and strengthen the muscle tone in the airway. In addition, these drugs reduce REM sleep, a time when SDB tends to be worse. Protriptyline (Vivactil) and more recently fluoxetine (Prozac) are two examples of antidepressants that are sometimes used to treat SDB. However, these medications should be used only if specifically prescribed for the patient for this condition and only if the physician is closely following that patient's progress to avoid any negative side effects.

For central sleep apnea, sleep specialists initially try to correct underlying problems such as heart or neurologic disease. If such treatments are not successful, patients may respond to medications such as acetazolamide (Diamox) and theophylline (Theo-Dur, Theo-24), although it is uncommon for these medications to offer any substantial benefits in the long term.

CHAPTER SUMMARY

Although the exact risks of SDB currently are not well defined and are the focus of considerable research, for some patients SDB can be a serious disorder if left untreated. In SDB, sleep is very disturbed and the brain is deprived of oxygen at night, which can lead to memory problems, concentration problems, medical problems, and daytime sleepiness. One of the most serious consequences is falling asleep while driving. If you snore loudly or are experiencing daytime sleepiness, you should talk to your doctor about a sleep evaluation.

6) NARCOLEPSY

WHAT IS NARCOLEPSY?

Narcolepsy is a sleep disorder characterized primarily by irresistible sleepiness during the day. In addition, patients with narcolepsy may experience cataplexy, sleep paralysis, and hypnagogic hallucinations. These four symptoms make up the "narcolepsy tetrad."

Levels of sleepiness can be so drastic that individuals with narcolepsy may fall asleep unintentionally in the middle of a conversation, while driving, or while eating a meal. Sometimes patients are unable to remember much of what they do during the day because they are so sleepy. They may "black out" while driving a car, forget that they made certain phone calls, or forget that they performed specific chores. They have difficulty performing quality work during dull and monotonous activities. The sleepiness is sometimes alleviated by short naps. In fact, many patients with narcolepsy schedule 10- to 20-minute naps into their daily routine. As you might imagine, such a magnitude of sleepiness often has unwelcome consequences. Many patients with narcolepsy have difficulty keeping jobs, friends, and even romantic relationships. However, it is important to understand that narcolepsy is not a psychologic disorder. Patients with narcolepsy are not sleepy because they are lazy, bored, or unmotivated, but rather because they have a physiologic problem.

WHAT IS CATAPLEXY?

In addition to daytime sleepiness, about 70% of patients with narcolepsy experience cataplexy. Cataplexy is a sudden muscular weakness, total loss of muscle tone, or paralysis brought on by strong emo-

53

tions such as anger, fear, hearty laughter, or crying. Cataplectic attacks often involve weakness in a specific part of the body. Weakness in the lower facial muscles may cause a slurring of words. Weakness of the limbs may result in wobbly movements or the dropping of objects. If the attacks are more severe, patients with narcolepsy may become altogether limp and fall to the floor. Since these episodes are preceded by moments of emotional excitement, patients with narcolepsy often avoid certain situations that may bring on intense emotional reactions. Cataplectic attacks usually do not last more than a few minutes. Patients are conscious during the attacks and are aware of everything that is going on around them. The frequency of the attacks varies from patient to patient. In some patients with narcolepsy, cataplexy attacks may occur infrequently (once a month or less), whereas in others they may occur several times a day.

WHAT ARE THE OTHER SYMPTOMS OF THE NARCOLEPSY TETRAD?

Approximately 20% to 30% of patients with narcolepsy experience the full narcolepsy tetrad. The other two symptoms of the tetrad are sleep paralysis (experienced by 40% to 65%) and hypnagogic hallucinations (experienced by 50% to 70%). Sleep paralysis occurs just as the narcoleptic patient begins to fall asleep. The patient is paralyzed except for respiration and eye movements. Hypnagogic hallucinations are very vivid visual and auditory dreamlike phenomena that may occur at the same time as the sleep paralysis. The hallucinations are generally short-lived and end abruptly. Patients with narcolepsy may report "seeing things," which can range from simple geometric shapes to picturesque landscapes. Auditory hallucinations may involve a range of sounds, from music to human voices. The emotional qualities of hypnagogic hallucinations commonly involve intense fear and anxiety. Hallucinations involving prowlers or intruders are often reported. Indeed, both the sleep paralysis and the hypnagogic hallucinations can be very terrifying experiences. As a consequence, some patients learn to dread the experience of going to bed. Although these episodes are dreams, they seem very real to the person with narcolepsy.

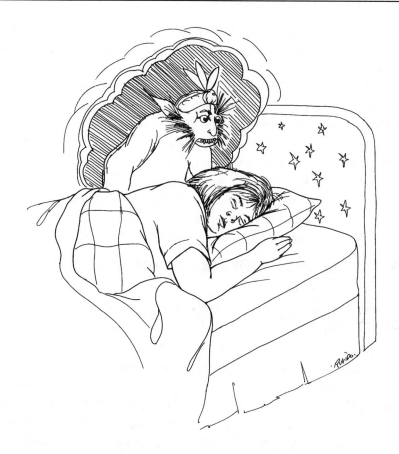

WHAT CAUSES THE SYMPTOMS OF NARCOLEPSY?

The exact cause of narcolepsy is not fully understood, although there is a strong genetic component to the disorder. Relatives of patients with narcolepsy are at a much greater risk for developing the disorder. Narcolepsy may involve both the central nervous system and the immune system. Recently, researchers have uncovered a link between narcolepsy and DR2, a human leukocyte antigen. Although there is no cure for narcolepsy at this time, recent discoveries such as this link help scientists to better understand the disorder.

Narcolepsy commonly begins sometime between the teenage years and young adulthood. The first symptom to appear is the day-

55

time sleepiness. Symptoms of cataplexy may not appear until several years later. It is believed that cataplexy, sleep paralysis, and hypnagogic hallucinations are the result of a partial activation of REM sleep while the person is still awake. Cataplexy is very much like the paralysis experienced during REM sleep. The difference is that this partial activation of REM sleep during cataplexy involuntarily intrudes on wakefulness. The brain waves during a cataplectic attack reveal a pattern suggesting wakefulness.

Sleep paralysis is similar to cataplexy, although the patient with narcolepsy is usually in bed. Hypnagogic hallucinations can be viewed as manifestations of REM sleep. It is as if while lying in bed, a dream inappropriately begins while the person is still conscious.

WHAT HAPPENS TO THE PERSON WITH NARCOLEPSY DURING SLEEP?

Patients with narcolepsy tend to have "lighter" sleep at night and wake up more frequently than most individuals. They also tend to have excessive periodic limb movements (see Chapter 7) during sleep. However, these phenomena don't altogether explain the severe daytime sleepiness seen in narcolepsy. Besides, some patients with narcolepsy get plenty of good quality sleep at night and still find themselves very sleepy during the day. Rather, narcolepsy is often viewed as a disorder of rapid eye movement (REM) sleep or as an imbalance between the physiologic mechanisms that control sleep and wake.

As explained in Chapter 2, when we fall asleep at night, most of us go directly into non–rapid eye movement (NREM) sleep. After approximately an hour and a half of NREM sleep, we then enter REM sleep. On the other hand, patients with narcolepsy often enter REM sleep as soon as they fall asleep, that is, they have sleep onset REM periods. When patients with narcolepsy fall asleep unintentionally during the day, they also may enter REM sleep right away. This is why narcolepsy is considered a disorder of REM sleep. In fact, it is believed that cataplexy, as well as sleep paralysis and hypnagogic hallucinations, is caused by the motor inhibition mechanism of REM sleep breaking through into the waking state. However, patients with narcolepsy do not always enter REM sleep immediately. They may enter NREM sleep first, just as most of us do. For this reason some researchers and doctors prefer to conceptualize narcolepsy as an imbalance in the brain's chemical systems that regulate sleep and wakefulness.

When the sleep of a patient with narcolepsy is recorded, in addition to the sleep onset REM period, we see multiple awakenings and increased stage 1 (light) sleep. Recordings conducted for 24 hours indicate that the total sleep time patients with narcolepsy get within the 24-hour period is not different from the total sleep time of individuals without narcolepsy. However, in this patient, the sleep occurs in more than one nighttime episode. The patient tends to fall asleep when awake and to wake up when asleep because he has difficulty conserving whichever state he is in.

HOW COMMON IS NARCOLEPSY?

Narcolepsy is found in about 6 out of every 1000 people in the world. It has been estimated that in the United States about 250,000 people have narcolepsy. In fact, in the United States, narcolepsy is more common than multiple sclerosis.

HOW DOES THE SLEEP SPECIALIST DETERMINE IF I HAVE NARCOLEPSY?

A sleep specialist who suspects that you may have narcolepsy will want to ask you questions about your sleep patterns and feelings of sleepiness. In addition to general sleep questions (see Chapter 12), the doctor will ask questions specifically related to the symptoms of narcolepsy. For example, you might be asked about whether you ever experience muscular weakness, and if so, what triggers these experiences.

You will then need to spend at least one night sleeping in the sleep clinic. The only way to make an objective diagnosis of narcolepsy is to record sleep and to observe if sleep onset REM periods occur. In addition, you will be asked to take a second sleep test during the day following your night recording, either a multiple sleep latency test (MSLT) (Fig. 6-1) or a maintenance of wakefulness test (MWT). Both tests measure how sleepy you are during the day. During the MSLT, you will be asked to go to sleep four to five times during the day, at 2-hour intervals. During the MWT, you will be asked to sit in a room with the lights turned off and try to stay awake. With both of these tests, the amount of sleepiness you experience can be objectively measured.

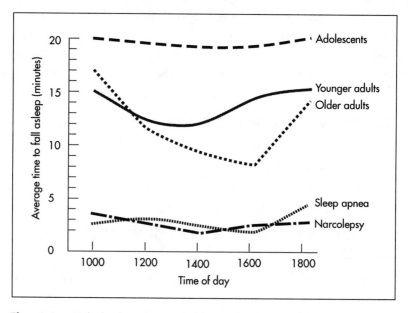

Fig. 6-1 Multiple sleep latency test. (Modified from Dement WC, Seidel W, Carskadon M: Daytime alertness, insomnia and benzodiazepines, *Sleep* 5:S28-S54, 1982.)

HOW IS NARCOLEPSY TREATED?

Narcolepsy cannot be cured. However, the symptoms of narcolepsy can be treated and brought under control. The sleepiness of narcolepsy can be treated with medications that help to keep you awake. The cataplexy is usually treated with tricyclic antidepressants (not for the antidepressing action, but because these drugs have the physical effect of reducing REM sleep). Since some of the drugs used to treat narcolepsy can become addicting, it is extremely important to see your doctor on a regular basis.

Your doctor may also recommend that you take brief voluntary naps throughout the day to help you stay vigilant and that you avoid alcohol, which can make all the symptoms worse. If you find that you need further emotional support, you may wish to get in touch with a psychotherapist and/or join support groups that have been established just for patients with narcolepsy (see Chapter 12 for list of organizations).

7) PERIODIC LIMB MOVEMENTS IN SLEEP

Periodic limb movements in sleep (PLMS) is a disorder in which the limbs (primarily the legs) twitch or jerk every 20 to 40 seconds during sleep (Fig. 7-1). This disorder was previously called nocturnal myoclonus. Each movement lasts between half a second to five seconds and can involve the big toe, ankle, knee, and sometimes the hip. Some patients also experience jerking of the arms. Most jerks cause a brief awakening; as if every time you fell asleep, someone shook you just enough to wake you again. PLMS is not to be confused with hypnic jerks (sensation of falling), which only occur at sleep onset and are considered normal (see Chapter 10).

HOW IS A DIAGNOSIS OF PERIODIC LIMB MOVEMENTS IN SLEEP MADE?

As part of the normal clinical workup, leg movements are recorded during sleep. Sensors are placed over the tibialis muscle on the calf of each leg. The number of times you kick your legs during each hour of sleep is counted. This is called the myoclonus index. If you kick your legs at least 5 times for every hour of sleep (that is, if the myoclonus index ≥ 5), with each kick causing an awakening, then the diagnosis of PLMS is made.

The kicks generally occur in the lighter stages of sleep, for example, stage 1 or stage 2 sleep. Therefore people who kick often have difficulty falling asleep, since each time they begin to enter stage 1 or

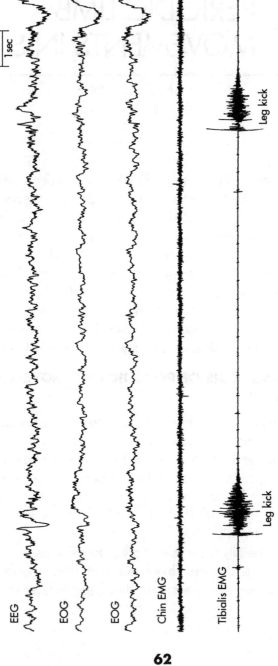

Fig. 7-1 A leg kick in a person with periodic limb movements in sleep (PLMS). *EEG*, electroencephalograph or brain waves; *EOG*, electro-oculograph or eye movements; *EMG*, electromyograph or muscle tension of the chin; *EMG*, muscle tension of the tibialis muscle of the leg.

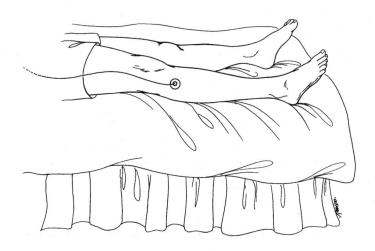

stage 2 sleep, their leg movements wake them up. It is less common to see kicks during REM sleep or during the deeper stages of sleep.

The number of kicks vary from night to night, so sometimes two nights of recording are necessary. The kicks can occur in one leg at a time, in both legs together, or alternate from one leg to the other.

Although PLMS is a sleep disorder of its own, it is not unusual to also find it in patients who have sleep disordered breathing (see Chapter 5) or narcolepsy (see Chapter 6). Periodic limb movements in sleep also has been associated with diabetes, renal disease, anemia, uremia, chronic lung disease, leukemia, and arthritis. Certain medications can make PLMS worse, such as certain tricyclic antidepressants (a class of drug used to treat depression).

WHAT SYMPTOMS ARE ASSOCIATED WITH PERIODIC LIMB MOVEMENTS IN SLEEP?

Patients with PLMS often complain of sleep onset insomnia because as soon as they relax enough to fall asleep, their legs begin to jerk, thus waking them again. Many patients are unaware that they kick but are aware of difficulty falling asleep. Patients who wake up numerous times during the night might also experience excessive daytime sleepiness. Some patients with PLMS also complain of feeling restless at night, whereas some complain of having extremely cold feet.

Individuals with PLMS are reported to sleep about an hour less per night than people without periodic limb movements in sleep. Interestingly, the prevalence of periodic limb movements in sleep is not higher in insomniac patients than those without insomnia.

It is often useful to have your bed partner accompany you to the doctor's office, since the bed partner may be more aware than you, the patient, are about the kicking and leg twitches during sleep. In fact, bed partners are often sleeping in separate beds to avoid being kicked all night long.

WHAT IF MY LEGS ARE RESTLESS DURING THE DAY?

A related disturbance, restless legs syndrome (RLS) is associated with uncomfortable, creepy, crawling sensations in the lower legs, feet, or thighs that result in an irresistible urge to move the limbs. Sometimes these sensations are described as "pins and needles" in the leg. These sensations are called dysesthesias or paresthesias. These sensations generally occur when you are relaxed or resting and often

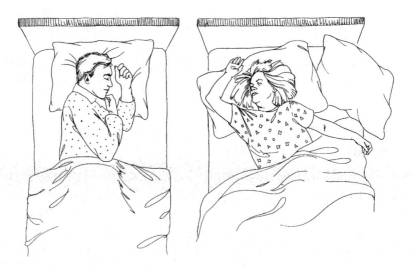

interfere with falling asleep. Some patients experience the same sensations when they wake up at night, and find themselves walking or rubbing their legs to try to relieve the uncomfortable feelings.

Restless legs syndrome is frequently seen in patients with uremia, kidney failure, rheumatoid arthritis, or in pregnant women. Drinking large amounts of caffeine may make the symptoms worse, as may being overly tired and exposure to a very cold or very warm environment. Typically, RLS begins in the third decade of life, but commonly gets worse with age. Often RLS is hereditary.

Almost all patients with RLS have periodic limb movements in sleep, but not all patients with periodic limb movements in sleep have restless legs syndrome. Patients with RLS may also complain of insomnia or of excessive daytime sleepiness.

WHAT CAUSES PERIODIC LIMB MOVEMENTS IN SLEEP, AND CAN IT BE TREATED?

The cause of periodic limb movements in sleep is unknown. Some doctors have suggested that the movements are caused by reactions in the brain, whereas others suggest it might originate in the spinal cord or may be associated with circulatory problems.

Periodic limb movements in sleep is treatable with several different medications. Unfortunately, since we do not know what causes the leg movements, it is sometimes difficult to know how best to treat it. Not all medications work in all people so you and your doctor may need to try different treatments before you find the one that works best for you.

The different medications recommended include certain sleeping pills, certain types of pain killers, and some of the drugs used in Parkinson's disease (although the two disorders are not related).

The most common sleeping pills used to treat PLMS are some of the benzodiazepines such as clonazepam (Klonopin) or temazepam (Restoril). These drugs reduce the number of awakenings at night, but have little effect on the number of leg jerks. Therefore the symptom of insomnia disappears but the symptoms of leg movements do not, or in other words, you still kick your legs but it no longer wakes you up.

The pain killers used to treat PLMS include drugs with opiates (such as Tylenol with codeine). These drugs reduce the number of leg kicks, but do not always reduce all the awakenings. In other words, you may stop kicking, but you may still wake up periodically. These drugs also are potentially addictive and only should be used at the lowest possible dose and only if prescribed by your physician.

The third class of drugs used to treat PLMS are the dopaminergic drugs such as L-dopa (for example, Sinemet). These are the same drugs used to treat Parkinson's disease. L-dopa is given at bedtime and again halfway through the night or in one slow release pill. Although these drugs eliminate both the leg kicks and the awakenings, there are some serious potential side effects. Some patients experience sudden onset of leg kicks during the day (that is, daytime rebound) as the L-dopa leaves their body. In younger patients there may also be the potential of developing tardive dyskinesia. No follow-up studies have yet been completed to understand the long-term effect of taking these drugs.

HOW COMMON ARE PERIODIC LIMB MOVEMENTS IN SLEEP AND RESTLESS LEGS SYNDROME?

Diagnosis for both periodic limb movements in sleep and restless legs syndrome usually is made when the patient is middle-aged, since that is often the first time the patient reports symptoms to his or her doctor. However, many patients report having had the same sensations as adolescents and even as children. Doctors have suggested that this disorder may be inherited, because it does seem to run in families.

The prevalence of PLMS in young and middle-aged adults has not been fully established, although the prevalence seems to increase with age. Among patients seen in sleep disorders clinics, about 17% of those complaining of insomnia and 11% of those complaining of excessive daytime sleepiness are diagnosed with periodic limb movements in sleep. It has been estimated that PLMS is found in 5% of adults 30 to 50 years old and 29% of adults over the age of 50. However in the elderly, this condition is extremely common, with over 40% having at least 5 leg kicks per hour of sleep.

Features of Periodic Limb Movements in Sleep

—Leg kicks every 20 to 40 seconds
—Duration of 0.5 to 5 seconds
—Complaints of
  • Insomnia
  • excessive sleepiness
  • restless legs
  • cold or hot feet
  • uncomfortable sensations in the legs

8) CIRCADIAN RHYTHMS

All of us have biologic rhythms that fluctuate approximately every 24 hours. These are called our circadian rhythms. The sleep/wake cycle is one example of a circadian rhythm. Core body temperature and certain hormones (such as cortisol and prolactin) also fluctuate in a circadian rhythm. The circadian rhythms are controlled by the suprachiasmatic nucleus (SCN), which is located in the anterior hypothalamus in the brain. If the SCN were surgically removed, sleep would occur as many brief naps during the day and night, rather than as one long sleep period at night.

Circadian rhythms are measured by their cycle length, called tau, amplitude (lowest point versus highest point of the rhythm), and phase (clock time such as hour of greatest alertness). The circadian rhythms interact with each other; for example core body temperature interacts with the sleep/wake cycle (Fig. 8-1). The core body temperature is not always 98.6° F. It can naturally go as high as 100° F in the afternoon and as low as 96° F in the early morning hours right before we wake up. We become sleepy whenever our body temperature begins to drop (in the afternoon after it hits its zenith) and again in the evening. This explains why we often feel more tired in the afternoon and again at night.

Our internal rhythms are synchronized (aligned) with external rhythms (that is, the environment) by cues such as light. These cues are called zeitgebers ("time-givers"). The zeitgeber light enters the retina of the eye and travels through the retinohypothalamic tract to the SCN. As the intensity of light changes (sunrise through sunset), our

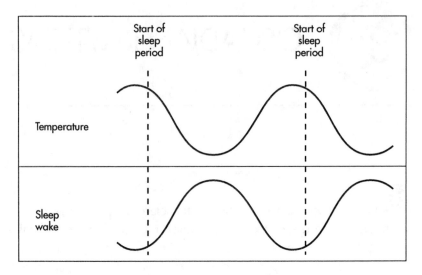

Fig. 8-1 Temperature cycle and sleep cycle.

sleep/wake cycle also changes. If we had no time cues (clocks) and no light cues (sunlight) and could choose our own sleep/wake cycles, our circadian rhythms would run approximately 25 hours, rather than the clock time of 24 hours. For us to stay in tune with the sun/moon, light/dark cycle, we must therefore shorten our rhythms by 1 hour each day by exposing ourselves to bright light (sunlight). This is called phase-advancement. Being exposed to bright light at different times of the cycle causes our rhythms to move earlier (phase-advance) or move later (phase-delay).

Sometimes our circadian rhythms become desynchronized. For example, when we travel to a different time zone our sleep/wake cycle is forced to change, but our temperature cycle is still on our old schedule. We then have difficulty sleeping until our temperature cycle has adjusted to the new time zone. Because our clocks run at 25 hours, it is harder for our clocks to shorten the time, that is, phase advance. It is easier to lengthen the clock time (phase-delay). For this reason, it is easier to travel from east to west since that makes our days longer, which is more in line with our longer body clocks.

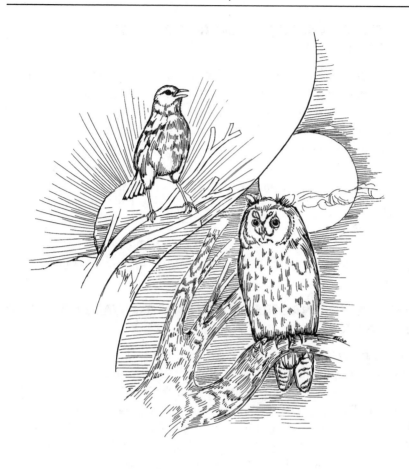

Conversely, it is harder to travel from west to east since that shortens our day and forces us to go to bed earlier.

Some people's rhythms might be a little shorter or longer than 24 hours. These people are often known as "morning types" or larks, or as "evening types" or owls. Larks like to go to bed early and wake up early; they function best in the morning. Owls like to go to bed late and wake up late; they function best in the evening. However, for some owls or larks this type of circadian rhythm can present problems.

WHEN ARE CIRCADIAN RHYTHM DISORDERS A PROBLEM?

Circadian rhythm disturbances result from a mismatch between the body clock and the environment. Your need to sleep does not match your social or environmental situation, or more specifically, does not match the light/dark cycle. For some people this mismatch is not a problem. However, for others, this mismatch interferes with their ability to sleep when they want to or to be alert when they need to be. For those people, insomnia, hypersomnia, sleepiness, and fatigue result in significant discomfort and impairment. For this reason, the diagnosis of a circadian rhythm disorder is based on a careful study of the patient's sleep history and on an examination of the patient's circadian patterns of sleep and wake, of napping, of alertness, and of behavior.

WHY ARE TEENAGERS SO DIFFICULT TO WAKE UP IN THE MORNING?

As we progress from infancy to old age, our rhythms shift. In late adolescence our rhythms begin to phase delay. This means that college-age teenagers will not get sleepy until the early morning hours (for example, 1:00 or 2:00 in the morning). If allowed to sleep, they will sleep for 8 or 9 hours, but that means they do not wake up until 10:00 or 11:00 in the morning. As we continue to age, our rhythm begins to advance, that is, we begin to get sleepier earlier and wake up earlier, and thus we shift back to being sleepy around 10:00 PM or 11:00 PM and waking up at about 7:00 AM. However, some people get stuck in the delayed phase and continue to go to sleep late and wake up late. This is called a delayed sleep phase syndrome (see Fig. 8-2).

WHAT ARE THE SYMPTOMS OF DELAYED SLEEP PHASE SYNDROME?

People with delayed sleep phase may be extreme versions of the owls or night people. Many owls have learned to enjoy their evening "alertness" and have little desire to change their pattern. Individuals

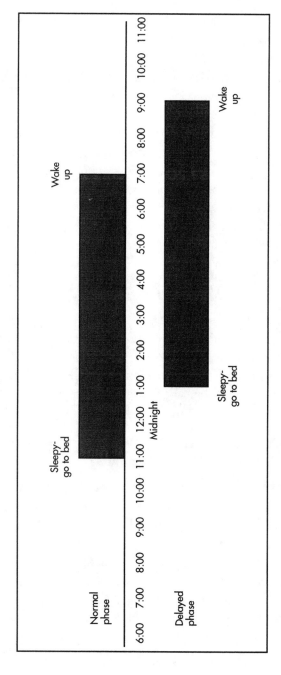

Fig. 8-2 Delayed sleep phase syndrome.

with delayed sleep phase syndrome often choose careers that allow them to set their own schedules, such as free-lance writing.

However, for those not able to adjust their lifestyle, delayed sleep phase syndrome becomes a serious sleep disorder. People with this disorder often complain of insomnia or difficulty falling asleep if they try to get to sleep at a more acceptable hour, such as 11:00 PM. In the morning they are very difficult to arouse, and they often are late for early morning appointments. In addition, when they are forced to get up early, they experience daytime sleepiness because they do not get enough sleep at night and are awake during their sleepy phase.

At this time the most effective treatment for delayed sleep phase syndrome is bright-light therapy. As explained earlier, bright light is the best synchronizer of the circadian rhythms. Bright light exposure in the early morning hours will phase advance the delayed rhythm, that is, cause the person to become sleepy earlier in the night. This treatment should be done in consultation with your physician or with a sleep disorders specialist. People with delayed sleep phase syndrome should be encouraged to remove blinds and curtains from their windows, which would allow the sunlight to pour into their bedrooms in the morning when they should arise.

WHY IS MY GRANDFATHER ALWAYS WAKING UP AT 3:00 OR 4:00 IN THE MORNING?

As mentioned previously, as we age our rhythm advances. This means that as we get older, we get sleepy earlier and earlier in the evening. We usually still sleep for 7 to 8 hours, but if we go to sleep at 7:00 or 8:00 in the evening, that means we wake up at 3:00 or 4:00 in the morning. This is called advanced sleep phase syndrome (Fig. 8-3). People with advanced sleep phase syndrome still get the same amount of sleep, but their rhythm is shifted forward into the evening. These people are the extreme larks because they are most alert in the morning.

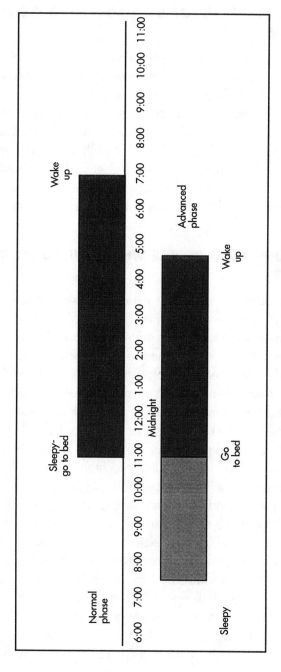

Fig. 8-3 Advanced sleep phase syndrome.

WHAT ARE THE SYMPTOMS OF ADVANCED SLEEP PHASE SYNDROME?

People with advanced sleep phase syndrome complain of sleep maintenance insomnia, that is, they wake up in the early morning hours and cannot fall back to sleep. Some individuals also may complain of daytime sleepiness because they start getting sleepy in the afternoon. This condition is less common than delayed sleep phase syndrome and is more prevalent in the elderly (see Chapter 11). The best treatment for advanced sleep phase syndrome is also bright light therapy, but this time the light exposure should occur in the evening, which will delay the rhythm or make you sleepier later in the evening.

WHAT HAPPENS TO PEOPLE WHO HAVE TO WORK AT NIGHT?

Shift work problems occur when the circadian sleep-wake rhythm is in conflict with your work schedule. Nearly 25% of Americans have jobs that require them to work at night. There are different patterns of shift work including rotating schedules and more or less permanent evening and night schedules. Rotating schedules, particularly rapidly shifting schedules, often cause problems because it is extremely difficult for the body to constantly readjust its clock. It is even more difficult when the shift worker tries to live on a "normal" schedule on his or her day off. Even if the worker can adjust his circadian system to the work schedule, he is then out of synchrony with the rhythm of his family and friends when he's not working. Shift workers are constantly sleep deprived and therefore sleepy. The sleepiness results in impaired performance and increased risk of accidents; more bodily complaints; poor morale; and excessive use of sleeping pills, stimulants, and alcohol. Shift work schedules may have played a role in human errors that contributed to the disasters at Three Mile Island, Chernobyl, and the Challenger lift-off explosion.

No ideal solutions exist for managing shift work problems. There is much variation in people's ability to adjust to these shift work schedules. Self-selection or "survival of the fittest" may be involved. Since

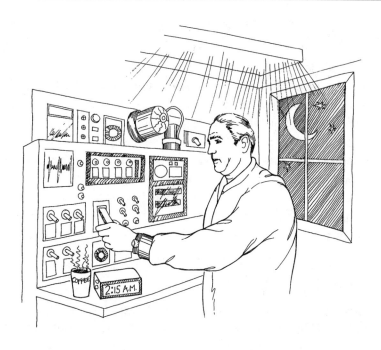

the biologic clock tends to have a natural cycle of 25 hours, it is easier to shift in a clockwise direction, that is, from morning shift to afternoon shift to evening shift to graveyard shift, rather than from night to evening, etc. Older people have a more difficult time adjusting to shift work. Appropriate exposure to bright lights and darkness may help shift workers move their rhythms. This might involve installing bright lights in the work place, using dark sunglasses on the way home, and installing blackout curtains at home to maintain darkness during the day. Naps may also be useful in reducing sleep loss. Small amounts of coffee may help shift workers stay alert early in the shift, but should be avoided near the end of the shift when it could interfere with daytime sleep.

HOW DO I GET OVER JET LAG?

When we travel across different time zones, our bodies become jet lagged. This means that although we are physically in a new

77

time zone, our bodies still want to wake, sleep, eat, etc. at our old time zone. On its own, it would take the body clock several days (or longer depending on how many time zones you cross) to adjust. As described earlier, however, the internal body clock can be reset more quickly using bright light exposure. By exposing ourselves to bright light (for example, being in sunlight without sunglasses, since the light enters through the eyes) and to darkness during appropriate times, we can begin to shift the internal body clock within a day and achieve complete adaptation within about 3 days.

Dr. Roger Cole and Henry Savage, CME, have developed a light exposure calculator, which they have agreed to reproduce here. The calculator shows you which times of day to be exposed to bright light and which times to avoid bright light.

For eastbound trips that cross 1 to 10 time zones, the calculator shows you the local time at your point of destination at which you should begin exposing yourself (your eyes) to daylight. The ideal duration of exposure is about 4 hours. You should avoid light for about 8 hours before the local destination time. If possible, this is the best time to sleep or stay indoors. If you must be outdoors, wear dark sunglasses. On the second day, repeat the procedure but start 2 hours *earlier*. Each day, shift another 2 hours earlier until you are adjusted to the local time.

For westbound trips, or if you cross more than 11 to 12 time zones, the calculator shows the local time at your point of destination at which you should end your bright light exposure. Avoid light after the time shown. Each day, shift your times of light and dark 2 hours *later*, until you are adjusted.

For example, if you are traveling from New York to London, you are traveling east across five time zones. According to the calculator, on your first day in London, you would avoid light before 10:00 AM and try to stay outdoors for at least 4 hours after 10:00 AM. On the second day, you would avoid light before 8:00 AM and try to be outdoors after 8:00 AM.

Light Exposure Calculator

Time Zones Crossed		Local Time at Destination	
2E	Avoid light before→	7:00 am	←Get light after
3E	Avoid light before→	8:00 am	←Get light after
4E	Avoid light before→	9:00 am	←Get light after
5E	Avoid light before→	10:00 am	←Get light after
6E	Avoid light before→	11:00 am	←Get light after
7E	Avoid light before→	12:00 pm	←Get light after
8E	Avoid light before→	1:00 pm	←Get light after
9E	Avoid light before→	2:00 pm	←Get light after
10E	Avoid light before→	3:00 pm	←Get light after
11E	Get light before→	4:00 pm	←Avoid light after
12E/W	Get light before→	5:00 pm	←Avoid light after
11W	Get light before→	6:00 pm	←Avoid light after
10W	Get light before→	7:00 pm	←Avoid light after
9W	Get light before→	8:00 pm	←Avoid light after
8W	Get light before→	9:00 pm	←Avoid light after
7W	Get light before→	10:00 pm	←Avoid light after
6W	Get light before→	11:00 pm	←Avoid light after
5W	Get light before→	12:00 am	←Avoid light after
4W	Get light before→	1:00 am	←Avoid light after
3W	Get light before→	2:00 am	←Avoid light after
2W	Get light before→	3:00 am	←Avoid light after

E, East; *W*, west.
From Cole R, Savage H: New light on jet lag, 1995, Circadian Solutions.

WHAT IS MELATONIN?

There is much on-going research into a hormone called melatonin, which is secreted by the pineal gland in the brain. Melatonin may turn out to be very effective for treating circadian rhythms disorders, such as delayed or advanced sleep phase syndrome or jet lag, and may also be effective as a sleeping aid. Although the research is very promising, at the time of this writing, melatonin treatment has not been approved by the Federal Drug Administration.

9) SLEEP OF CHILDREN

HOW DO SLEEP/WAKE PATTERNS DEVELOP IN INFANTS?

Sleep and wake patterns have been traced to babies still in the womb. At approximately 36 weeks of gestational age, the preterm infant begins to spend regular times asleep and awake. In the first 6 months of life, the infant's sleep pattern continues to develop into distinct sleep periods and wake periods. Studies at Stanford University have shown that at 3 weeks of age, infants sleep an average of 212 minutes before waking. By 6 months of age, they are sleeping an average of 358 minutes. Over the first 6 months, sleep begins to consolidate and follow the light (day)/dark (night) cycle.

By 6 months, most infants' longest sleep period is at night, between 6:00 PM and 6:00 AM. However, many infants may not have regular sleep periods. Some research studies have shown that about one in every four infants still wakes up at night after the age of 1 year. Remember also that each child is different. Just because your older child slept through the night at 6 months it does not mean that your second child will do the same thing.

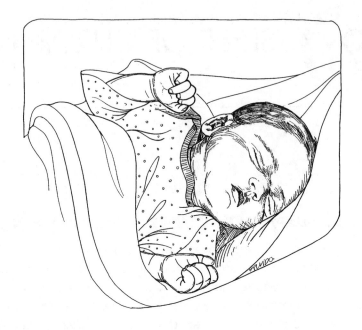

HOW DOES SLEEP CHANGE AS CHILDREN GROW?

Between the ages of 6 and 12 years, sleep needs continue to change, with the total sleep time decreasing as the amount of time spent in each stage of non–rapid eye movement (NREM) and rapid eye movement (REM) sleep decreases. In general, children in this age range spend 8 to 9.5 hours in bed, falling asleep within 20 minutes.

Dr. Mary Carskadon and her colleagues have studied sleep in preadolescents (ages 7 to 9 years) and adolescents. The preadolescents slept around 9 hours and were very alert during the day. Adolescents, who were going through physical and hormonal changes, slept about the same amount of time, indicating that the need to sleep did not decrease with age. On the other hand, at about age 13, adolescents became more sleepy during the day, suggesting that they may actually need more sleep at night. However, perhaps because of increased social activities and increased homework, these adolescents go to bed later and therefore get less sleep than they need.

HOW MUCH SLEEP DO CHILDREN NEED?

Sleep needs change dramatically from newborns to toddlers to children to young adults. Even more than in older individuals, there is much individual difference in how much sleep children need and at which point they give up their naps and begin sleeping through the night. As children grow, the amount of sleep needed decreases as does the depth of sleep. At the age of 4 or 5 years, as they begin to give up their naps, the total time children sleep is reduced. For about 25% of 2 year olds and 10% to 15% of 4-to-5 year old children, problems with waking up at night begin to develop.

On average most children need 11 to 12 hours of sleep. It is especially difficult for parents to determine how much sleep a child needs. In children, not sleeping enough may not manifest itself in daytime sleepiness but rather in the child being irritable, unable to pay attention or concentrate, and in emotional outbursts (for example, throwing tantrums).

As the child continues to grow, the total sleep time needed continues to decrease until around puberty. Research shows that most teenagers still need about 10 hours of sleep, although few adolescents get that much. However, at this age, the circadian rhythms begin

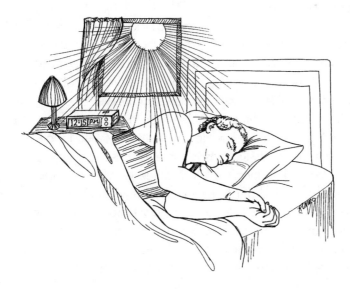

to phase delay, so that most teenagers get sleepier later in the night and awaken later in the morning (see Chapter 8).

WHY DO SOME CHILDREN HAVE TROUBLE FALLING ASLEEP?

Many of us have bedtime memories dating back to when we were children. Perhaps we didn't want to go to bed because we were scared of the dark. Maybe we were afraid of monsters hiding under the bed or were still frightened by the vivid images from the previous night's terrifying nightmare. It is not at all uncommon for children to have occasional nightmares and fears that surface at bedtime.

Children often experience anxiety during emotionally sensitive periods in their lives. Times commonly cited as potentially distressing for a child include the first days of daycare or nursery school. You may have seen a young child, perhaps your own, experience some type of separation anxiety as they're left off at school. Children may also feel anxious about certain events related to their newly discovered sexuality, such as masturbation and toilet training. Such anxieties often surface at bedtime, when the child is lying quietly in bed. Monsters, strange noises, and ambiguous fears may be manifestations of these anxieties.

As a consequence, children may have trouble falling asleep. They may get out of bed and tell you that they are scared or ask for another bedtime story. Perhaps they may resist going to bed altogether or may refuse to sleep alone. Again, these are normal consequences usually rooted in the normal anxieties experienced by small children.

Often these bedtime difficulties can be resolved without professional assistance. During the day, parents may wish to talk with their children about the issues responsible for their anxiety. Sometimes some simple reassurance is all that is needed. For example, children might need to hear that Mommy or Daddy will indeed return to pick them up from school or daycare. A few extra minutes comforting a child at bedtime may also provide him or her with the needed security for a peaceful bedtime (parents should not spend more than a few extra minutes with their child in most cases, since this may disrupt the child's normal sleep schedule). Consistent bedtimes are important for the child who has difficulty going to sleep.

However, other times a child may need more than a little reassurance. Particularly if a child's fear is deep-rooted, or if a child is resistant to the parent's attempts at communication during the day, the anxieties may be more difficult to diffuse. In some cases the fears at night are so great, and the disturbances from sleep so frequent and persistent, that a visit to a doctor trained in pediatric sleep disturbances may be called for.

WHAT DO THE SLEEP EXPERTS SAY ABOUT DEALING WITH CHILDREN'S SLEEP COMPLAINTS?

Dr. Richard Ferber is one of the, if not *the*, world's experts on how to deal with sleep problems in children. His book, *Solve Your Child's Sleep Problems,** is a good resource for any parent whose young child has difficulty sleeping. Briefly, Dr. Ferber suggests that in the younger child, problems arise from bad habits forming around falling asleep both at the beginning of the night, as well as after waking up in the middle of the night, and with excessive feedings at night.

All infants and children wake up during the night. This is part of normal sleep behavior. The problem occurs when the child is unable to fall back to sleep. Some children may cry out when they wake up at night. For example, if the child is used to falling asleep with the parent in the room or in the parent's arms, then when they wake up in the middle of the night and find themselves in bed alone, they may have difficulty falling back to sleep. A child who always falls asleep having his back rubbed will later be unable to fall asleep without having his back rubbed. Another child who falls asleep being rocked in a chair may wake up when placed in her crib. A third child may fall asleep sucking a pacifier that falls out once the child is asleep. If that child wakes later in the night without the pacifier, he will cry and be unable to fall back to sleep until the pacifier is replaced. These types of behavioral sleep problems are easy to correct within a few weeks.

---

*Ferber R: *Solve your child's sleep problems*, New York, 1985, Simon & Schuster.

In the child who has graduated out of a crib and into a bed, problems are usually related to the parents' being inconsistent in setting limits. Nighttime fears may play a role in the child's sleep problems, but fears are usually a very small part of the problem. Problems in this age group are usually related to falling asleep at bedtime. This child asks for one more story, one more glass of water, etc. If the parent gives in to the child's request, the child learns to keep asking. It is of great importance to set appropriate and consistent limits for the children. Once the child understands the rules ("You get one glass of water and then it is time to go to sleep."), she is more likely to stick to them and go to sleep.

WHAT ARE SOME COMMON SLEEP PROBLEMS IN CHILDREN?

Some sleep disorders occur primarily in children. Sleepwalking, night terrors, and nightmares are common in children. These disorders are called parasomnias because they occur when the person is partially awake. Parasomnias are described in Chapter 10. Nocturnal enuresis or bedwetting, headbanging, and body rocking also are common in young children and are described in this chapter.

WHAT IS NOCTURNAL ENURESIS?

Nocturnal enuresis is the inability to control urination during the night. It usually occurs during the early hours of a child's sleep. Although many young children may wet their beds, this behavior usually diminishes considerably by 6 years of age. In fact, by 3 years of age approximately three quarters of all children remain dry at night. Nevertheless, up to 25% of 4 year olds and up to 10% of 8 year olds still wet their beds. In one research study, 1% of 18 year olds still experienced enuresis.

Enuresis, like insomnia, is described as a symptom rather than a disorder. Many different problems could cause enuresis. These would include urologic problems (for example, urinary tract infections), constipation, diabetes, and small bladders.

Sometimes the child is sleeping so deeply that she is unaware of the cues the full bladder is trying to send to her. Other studies have drawn a link between enuresis and various allergies, sleep apnea, and hyperthyroidism. In such cases, the bedwetting would go away once these primary medical conditions are treated. Stress (such as family problems or problems at school) can also bring about bouts of bedwetting.

Children with nocturnal enuresis may experience guilt, embarrassment, and shame. Anxiety may arise when a child attempts to keep this behavior a secret from friends and family. Parents may also experience a good deal of distress. They may feel as if their child is misbehaving or rebelling. The act of changing a child's pajamas and bed linens repeatedly may become aggravating and tiresome.

HOW IS NOCTURNAL ENURESIS TREATED?

It is an interesting fact that a surprisingly large number of parents of children with enuresis wet their own beds as children. This has led doctors and researchers to draw a link between enuresis and heredity. In fact, if both parents wet their beds, approximately 75% of the parent's children will wet their beds as well.

An evaluation for bedwetting includes a urine analysis and urine culture to rule out an infection. If an infection is present, it will be treated with antibiotics. If another medical problem is the cause of the bedwetting, the medical problem should be treated first. The bedwetting may then go away on its own.

When the bedwetting is not a result of a medical disorder, it is commonly treated with behavioral interventions. In persistent cases the behavioral treatments may be supplemented with medication such as imipramine. A promising technique is to reward a child for remaining dry throughout the night. These children often enjoy earning stickers that over time can earn them a new toy or a favorite dessert. It is very important to not punish children for bedwetting. Giving out rewards for a desired behavior is almost always more effective than punishing an undesirable behavior. Reinforcing the desired behavior with a reward is only effective if the child has had one or two dry nights and you know he is able to control himself once in a while. If the child has not had a dry night, it may mean that he is not yet able to control himself and trying to promise a reward will only frustrate him further.

Many children also benefit from exercises designed to teach bladder control. These include holding off urination for a set time despite the urge to urinate, and intentionally stopping and restarting the flow of urine. Such exercises help teach children to recognize and control the sensations associated with a full bladder. Lastly, some specialists recommend the use of enuresis alarms, which can be wired to a pad that rests on a child's bed. The alarm is activated when the pad becomes moist and awakens the child. Over time, the child will learn to associate the sensations preceding urination with waking up.

Consistency, patience, and support among parents are important components in the behavioral strategies for enuresis. These treatments do not work overnight and may in fact work more slowly than most parents and children desire. However, when carried out consistently, they show considerable promise. Treatment should begin and end within a supportive and encouraging environment. Parents who belittle, punish, and blame their children for bedwetting may only make matters worse. Children generally do not wet their beds deliberately. It is undesirable for all involved—children and parents.

WHAT ARE HEADBANGING AND BODY ROCKING?

During the night, some children may thrust their heads against their pillows or the bed's headboard, or rock back and forth on their hands and knees in a rhythmic manner. This may occur during all hours of the night. Many parents are relieved to learn that this is quite common among small children and is considered normal. It is thought that children find these behaviors soothing and comforting. Headbanging and body rocking usually disappear by 3 years of age.

However, there are cases in which parents should attend to these behaviors seriously. Children, particularly if they start after 2 years of age, may be engaging in headbanging to get their parents' attention. This may be an indicator of emotional distress and may be best handled by a psychotherapist. Children with developmental disabilities often injure themselves and may benefit from wearing a helmet or some type of protective padding both for the child and for the environment around the bed. If the headbanging is persistent and recurrent, you may want to take the child to see a neurologist for possible neurologic problems.

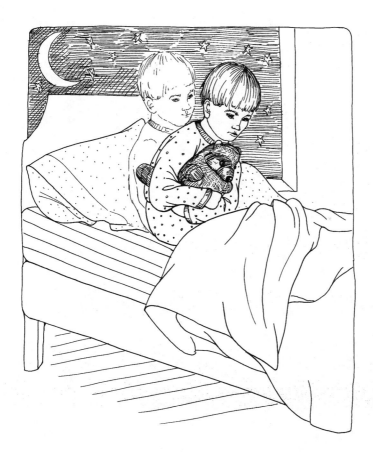

10) PARASOMNIAS

WHAT ARE PARASOMNIAS?

Parasomnias are intense, episodic physical events that occur during sleep or become worse during sleep. They occur primarily in children but might be found in adults as well. Some of these disorders occur in rapid eye movement (REM) sleep, whereas others occur secondary to a partial arousal (that is, awakening) during deep sleep. The partial arousal may mean that the normal mechanism that controls walking might be immature and causes walking while the rest of the brain is still asleep. Some of the more common parasomnias include sleepwalking, night terrors, nightmares, REM sleep behavior disorders, bruxism, sleep starts, and sleeptalking.

WHAT IS SLEEPWALKING?

Sleepwalkers are able to perform behaviors, such as walking, opening doors, climbing up or down stairs, while apparently sleeping. Sleepwalking generally occurs in the first third of the night. Contrary to popular belief, it does not occur during dream (REM) sleep, but rather during deep sleep (stages 3 and 4). Children will sometimes not even leave the bed, but rather will sit at the edge of the bed performing repetitive movements. When they do leave the bed, they walk with their eyes open and are usually able to avoid bumping into objects. However, sleepwalkers may walk through a window or fall down the stairs. They do not respond if spoken to and appear to be glassy-eyed or as if looking through people. Eventually they may find their way back to bed. If you wake them, they will be disoriented;

however, if left asleep, they can be led back to bed. Sleepwalkers are usually amnesic to the sleepwalking episode; that is, they have no memory or only a vague memory of the sleepwalking event in the morning. The episodes can last from several seconds to several minutes, although episodes as long as 1 hour have been reported. The average sleepwalking episode lasts about 6 minutes. It is unusual for more than one episode to happen in a night.

Sleepwalking in children is usually a condition that is not serious and one that the child will outgrow. The first episode of sleepwalking could appear as soon as the child learns to walk. However, sleepwalking is most common in children ages 4 to 8 years and usually disappears by the teenage years. Sleepwalking occurs in approximately 1% to 15% of children, occurring more often in boys than in girls. Often, sleepwalkers have other family members with a similar history of sleepwalking.

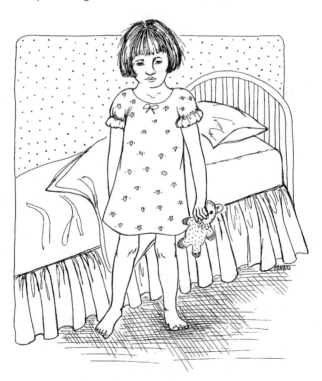

What to do if your Child Sleepwalks:

- Remove dangerous objects from surrounding areas.
- Keep doors and windows closed and locked.
- If necessary, move your child's room to the ground floor to keep her safe.
- Gently guide your child back to bed without waking him up.

From Masand R, Popli AP, Weilburg JB: Sleepwalking, *AM Fam Phys* 51:649-654, 1995.

In adults, sleepwalking is often associated with stress or psychologic problems. Usually adults have more sleepwalking episodes per year than children. In the elderly, sleepwalking should be examined very carefully to rule out side effects of medications, other medical illness, or dementia.

HOW IS SLEEPWALKING TREATED?

Most children outgrow sleepwalking without any intervention. Safety precautions can be taken, such as removing any dangerous or hazardous objects from the bedroom, having the sleepwalker sleep on the ground floor, locking windows, and placing a bell on the bedroom door to alert parents. Not sleeping enough at night or having irregular sleep schedules may bring on more sleepwalking episodes. It is therefore very important for the sleepwalker to get enough sleep at night and to go to bed at the same time each night.

Other treatments, particularly for adults, have included benzodiazepines (a type of sleeping pill) or other medications that suppress deep sleep, or psychotherapy. These treatments have varying degrees of success depending on the individual patient.

WHAT ARE NIGHT TERRORS?

Night terrors (also called pavor nocturnus) are also parasomnias. They generally occur during sleep in the first third of the night. During a night terror the person generally sits up in bed and screams. The episode can last several minutes, during which time the person experiences a racing heart, increased sweating, increased blood pressure, and dilated pupils. At the end of the episode the person lies down and returns to normal sleep; but if awakened, the person will be confused for 15 to 30 minutes. There is no memory of the event in the morning, therefore the night terror is much more frightening for the parent observing it than for the child experiencing it. Parents may try to comfort the child, but typically this only worsens the intensity of the terror. Instead of reaching out to be held, the child may resist parental affection and push them away. Children experiencing a night terror may appear confused with a strange facial expression and are typically unresponsive to their environment. Frequently, they show physiologic signs of anxiety (sweat, rapid heart rate).

Night terrors and sleepwalking frequently occur in the same person, although more children sleepwalk than have night terrors. Some children may outgrow one parasomnia and acquire another one.

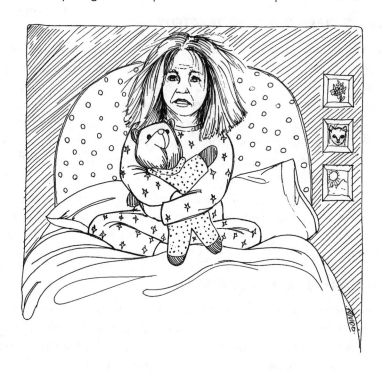

The prevalence of night terrors has been estimated to be about 1% to 6% in children and less than 1% in adults. It generally begins between the ages of 4 and 12 years and often goes away on its own. In adults it can begin between the ages of 20 and 30 years and may be associated with anxiety or post-traumatic stress disorder.

WHAT ARE NIGHTMARES?

Nightmares are frightening dreams that usually are very vivid and detailed. The content of the nightmare is frightening to the dreamer with common themes including being threatened, chased, hurt, or attacked. Although night terrors occur during non-rapid eye movement (NREM) sleep, nightmares occur during REM sleep. Since most of REM sleep occurs in the last third of the night (see Chapter 2), most nightmares also occur in the last third of the night.

Compared with night terrors, in which children frequently do not recall their nocturnal experiences on awakening, the memories of nightmares are often carried into the following day and may contribute to anxiety surrounding subsequent bedtimes. Memories of a terrifying nightmare can result in a child's resistance to going to sleep, to sleeping in his or her own bed, or to sleeping alone.

Children between the ages of 3 and 6 years are more likely to report their nightmares. Dr. David Foulkes, an expert on dreams, reports that at the younger ages children may have greater difficulty distinguishing between reality and dreams, and therefore will tell more about their nightmares than about other dreams. Between 30% and 50% of adults also report experiencing occasional nightmares. Nightmares are sometimes brought on by stressful events but generally are not considered sleep disorders.

HOW DO NIGHT TERRORS DIFFER FROM NIGHTMARES?

Night terrors and nightmares are two distinct nocturnal disturbances. Sleep terrors occur in deep sleep—usually in the first deep sleep cycle. In contrast, nightmares are thought to occur mainly in REM sleep. Thus sleep terrors commonly occur in the first third of the night during deep sleep; nightmares occur during the latter third of the night during REM sleep. (See Fig. 2-5.)

A child's state of confusion is another feature that differentiates night terrors from nightmares. Remember that a child who is having a night terror is really only partially awake. They tend not to make much sense when they speak and usually will not remember the event in the morning. A child who has had a nightmare is awake and does not appear as dazed and glassy-eyed. In addition, a child who is having a night terror will not be able to give a dream description to his or her parent, simply because no dream has preceded the event. Conversely, children are often able to describe their nightmares to their parents after awakening.

HOW ARE NIGHT TERRORS AND NIGHTMARES TREATED?

Usually night terrors and nightmares are not considered abnormal before 6 years of age. Parents who are aware of this and know how to handle such events are often relieved. However, night terrors and nightmares in children older than 6 may be suggestive of an emotional disturbance. This disturbance is not necessarily serious but may call for professional counseling. This is particularly true if the disturbances at night are frequent, violent, and their origin can be traced to a significant stressful event, such as a divorce or death in the family.

Clearly, a child in the midst of a night terror appears distressed. However, it can be distressing for the parents to watch their child scream and cry uncontrollably. Parents may instinctively want to reassure and comfort their child, both with words and with a hug. They may try to fully awaken their child, so as to terminate what may first appear to be a nightmare. They might want to comfort their child with words like, "It's only a dream." Parents often report that such efforts fail or only aggravate the night terror.

Experts believe that night terrors need to run their course, uninterrupted. They typically do not last more than 20 to 30 minutes, after which the child becomes sleepy and falls back to sleep. When parents attempt to awaken or comfort their child, they may be prolonging the duration of the night terror. Instead, parents should not attempt to intervene. Parents may wish, however, to go to their child's room to make sure he does not harm himself.

Children who seem to be excessively sleepy are also more prone to night terrors. Therefore it is important that children are getting enough sleep at night. In some cases, shifting a child's bedtime to an earlier hour may decrease the frequency of the night terrors. Parents should also attempt to keep their child's bedtime and wake-up time constant.

Since children typically do not remember a night terror the next morning, it is important for parents not to ridicule or tease their child about the previous night's experience. There really is no need for parents to mention it at all, for it may only make the child feel odd or foolish. If the child does ask about it, then it should be discussed in a manner so as not to embarrass him or her.

On the other hand, children should be comforted after they experience a nightmare. A parent's voice and affection may help the child come to the awareness that "it was just a dream" and that "it is over now." Typically a child who needs comfort will call out for it or will enter his or her parent's bedroom and want to talk about the nightmare. In contrast to the night terror, a child who has had a bad dream will reach out for his or her parent, wanting to be held.

If the frequency and intensity of the nightmares are severe, psychotherapy, behavioral techniques (such as hypnosis), or medication that reduces REM sleep would be beneficial. However, only rarely do nightmares require treatment.

WHAT IS RAPID EYE MOVEMENT SLEEP BEHAVIOR DISORDER?

Rapid eye movement sleep behavior disorder was only described for the first time in 1986, thus little is known about this disorder. REM sleep behavior disorder occurs when the muscle paralysis of REM sleep fails and the person experiences vigorous behavior during vivid dreaming. These behaviors, such as kicking, flailing, or punching, can result in injury both to the dreamer and to the bed partner. This

97

disorder is more common in older men in their 60s and 70s and may be associated with other neurologic diseases (such as dementia, Parkinson's disease, vascular disorders, multiple sclerosis, and alcohol withdrawal). The main complaint of the patient is injury during sleep, although some patients may complain of sleep disruptions. Since these behaviors occur during REM sleep, they generally begin about 90 minutes after the person falls asleep and can reoccur in the second half of the night when most REM sleep takes place. The disorder can get progressively worse. If you have these complaints, you should consult your doctor since REM sleep behavior disorder is treatable with low doses of a specific type of benzodiazepine, clonazepam (Klonopin).

WHAT IS BRUXISM?

Bruxism is teeth grinding during sleep. The bruxism generally occurs once per second for 5 seconds or longer. These episodes then repeat throughout the night. It is more common in children, although it has been estimated to affect between 10% to 20% of the adult population. As with many other sleep disorders, bruxism seems to run in families. Most people are not aware that they grind their teeth at night; more often it is discovered by the bed partner who can hear the loud grinding sound or by the dentist who finds that the teeth are being worn down. Patients may wake up with a sore jaw.

Bruxism generally gets better with age. It is thought to be related to stress and poor alignment of the teeth and jaw. It usually occurs in stage 2 sleep. Dentists treat bruxism in patients with special dental devices, sometimes in combination with relaxation training and biofeedback.

ARE THERE SLEEP BEHAVIORS THAT ARE CONSIDERED NORMAL?

Hypnic jerks, or sleep starts, happen to everyone. As you are falling asleep, this is the feeling that you are about to fall and you jerk yourself to stop your fall. This behavior is perfectly normal and needs no treatment.

Sleeptalking is also considered normal behavior that occurs most frequently in stage 2 sleep. There is no memory of this behavior, and it does not cause complaints of sleep disruptions. To reassure the child that she is not disclosing any secrets, it is important to convey to her that when she sleeptalks it is usually garbled and cannot be understood.

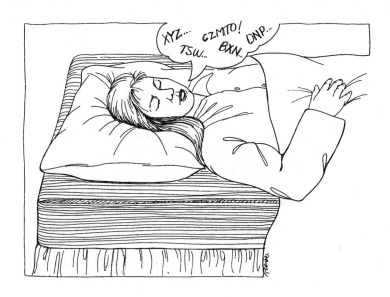

11) AGING AND SLEEP

As we age, many changes occur in our bodies. Parts of our body and mind begin to deteriorate and other parts slow down. But how many of these changes are part of normal aging and how many are pathologic conditions? In the area of sleep, some changes that occur are a result of normal aging and there are many others that are pathologic.

A second issue is the perception that older people have about their sleep. What is debilitating and disturbing to one older person, may feel normal to another. While one older person who sleeps only 6 hours a night might complain of trouble sleeping, another older person might adjust and have no complaints whatsoever.

WHAT DO OLDER PEOPLE REPORT ABOUT THEIR SLEEP?

Many surveys have been conducted about sleep in older people. Most older people report an increase in the number of awakenings experienced during the night, a decrease in total sleep time, an increase in the number of sleeping medications taken (particularly in women), an increase in daytime sleepiness, and consequently, an increase in napping behavior.

WHAT ARE THE NORMAL CHANGES THAT OCCUR IN SLEEP WITH AGE?

As reviewed in Chapter 2, our brain waves change with age, both in wake and in sleep. The alpha activity decreases, and in certain parts of the brain there is an increase in slow brain wave activity. In fact, slowing of the EEG is very common and has little pathologic significance in older, nondemented individuals.

Along with these changes in brain waves, there are some changes in sleep architecture (that is, our sleep cycles) and in quality of sleep. Sleep efficiency (how much we sleep when we are in bed) decreases to about 80%. The amounts of stage 1 and stage 2 sleep increase, and correspondingly, the amounts of stage 3 and stage 4 sleep (that is, deep sleep) decrease (Fig. 11-1). This decrease in deep sleep actually begins at around 20 years old. The time in our first REM period, which is 90 to 100 minutes in younger adults, also decreases.

Some of the sleep disturbances seen are secondary to specific conditions that are prevalent in elderly, such as nocturia, cardiovascular disease, pulmonary disease, diabetes, osteoarthritis, rheumatoid arthritis, and menopause. Other disturbances are secondary to medications (see list in Chapter 12).

Other changes also occur in sleep. There may be an increase in autonomic activity, for example, heart rate or blood pressure. Older people may become more sensitive to the environment. For example, they may hear more noises that will disturb their sleep. And, as mentioned in the following material and in Chapter 8, there are changes that occur in our biologic clocks or circadian rhythms.

IS INSOMNIA MORE COMMON IN OLDER PEOPLE?

Many studies have indicated that older people wake up more often during the night and have more complaints of insomnia. Two major problems exist with these conclusions.

The first problem is that many of these studies were done years ago, before laboratories had the knowledge to record respiration and leg movements. We now know that sleep disorders, such as sleep disordered breathing and periodic limb movements in sleep, will cause awakenings during the night that can lead to complaints of insomnia. Therefore many of those early results may really have been caused by these very common sleep disorders.

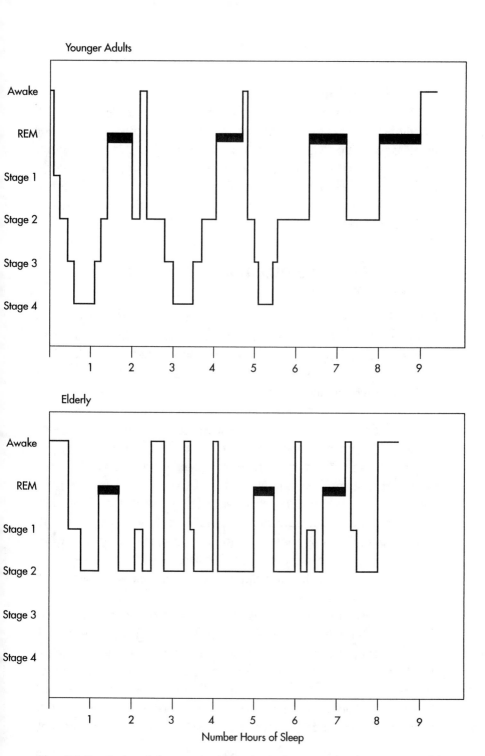

Fig. 11-1 Cycles of sleep in an older individual compared with a younger adult.

The second problem has to do with use of drugs and medical illnesses. Recent studies show that much of the poor sleep seen in the elderly is really caused by the large number of medical illness seen in this age group. Diseases such as nocturia (excessive nighttime urination), stomach and ulcer problems, heart disease, lung disease, diabetes, and chronic pain (from cancer, arthritis, etc.) all disturb sleep. The use of sleeping pills arises from the poor sleep caused by the medical disease. Therefore in the healthy aging adult, there should be no increase in the complaints of insomnia.

WHAT HAPPENS TO OUR BIOLOGIC CLOCKS AS WE AGE?

As we age, our biologic clocks or circadian rhythms are altered. The rhythm becomes more advanced, resulting in advanced sleep phase—a condition in which the older person gets sleepy early in the evening, goes to sleep, and then awakens 7 or 8 hours later, at 3:00 or 4:00 in the morning ("early to bed–early to rise") (see Chapter 8). Other changes in circadian rhythms result in more awakenings during the night and consequently, more naps taken during the day. In addition, older people have more difficulty adjusting to changes in time zones. Even if the older person with advanced sleep phase forces himself to stay up until 10:00 PM or 11:00 PM, his body will still wake up sometime between 3:00 AM and 5:00 AM (see Fig. 8-3). That means this individual only got 4 to 5 hours of sleep, less than he really needs. These individuals are then sleepy during the day. This has led to the misconception that older people *need* less sleep (that is, only 5 hours a night) and that it is normal for them to be sleepy during the day.

Circadian rhythm changes occur for several reasons. One reason may be that the change seen is part of the aging process itself. Other theories suggest that the changes are caused by changes in the lifestyle of the older person (such as loss of hearing, deterioration of eye sight). As mentioned in Chapter 8, light is the strongest cue for modifying circadian rhythms. As we age however, we may begin to spend less time outdoors, thus being exposed to less light. Patients who live in nursing homes are generally exposed to very little bright light; most of their days are spent indoors. In addition, eye disease such as cataracts, which are very common in older people, block out much of the light needed to modify the rhythms. It is believed that about 2 hours of bright light exposure is needed each day to modify or synchronize circadian rhythms. Yet one study by Dr. Scott Campbell and his colleagues and another study by my colleagues and I suggested that healthy elderly women were exposed to only 45 minutes of bright light per day, healthy elderly men were exposed to 90 minutes of bright light per day, Alzheimer's disease patients living at home were exposed to 30 minutes of bright light per day, and institutionalized nursing home patients were exposed to less than 2 minutes of bright light per day.

In summary, it seems that poor light exposure negatively affects sleep. More research is still needed on the ability of light to improve sleep and daytime functioning in the elderly. It may turn out to be a good nondrug treatment for some sleep problems.

WHAT ARE THE PATHOLOGIC CHANGES SEEN IN SLEEP?

Both sleep-disordered breathing (see Chapter 5) and periodic limb movements in sleep (see Chapter 7) have been proven to be very common in older people. Many of the symptoms attributed to aging, such as snoring, daytime sleepiness, hypertension, heart disease, and cognitive impairment are also symptoms of sleep-disordered breathing. Since these disorders are treatable, older people with symptoms severe enough to disturb their ability to function during the day should seek advice from their doctor.

HOW DOES MENOPAUSE AFFECT SLEEP?

Menopausal women have complaints of difficulty falling asleep, waking up often during the night, and feeling tired during the day. Some of these complaints are no different from complaints of all elderly adults, but some sleep problems can be attributed to the hormonal process. Hot flashes are believed to be related to estrogen levels and cause women to wake up over and over again during the night, with increased skin temperature, increased heart rate, and excessive sweating that requires a change of bedclothes and sheets. These repeated awakenings lead to daytime fatigue, irritability, and mood shifts. Women treated with estrogen have fewer hot flashes, wake up less often during the night, and have an easier time falling asleep.

WHAT HAPPENS TO SLEEP IN PATIENTS WITH DEMENTIA OR ALZHEIMER'S DISEASE?

Dementia is a progressive disorder of memory loss and confusion. One type of dementia is Alzheimer's disease. In dementia parts of the brain are deteriorating. This same deterioration leads to changes in our sleep.

Patients with dementia have no deep (stages 3 or 4) sleep and often experience decreases in REM sleep. Sleep efficiency is decreased and circadian rhythms are often reversed with patients waking up during the night and sleeping during the day. This reversal of wake and sleep, and the extreme sleep disruption seen at night, is the second leading cause of institutionalization in this country. (Incontinence is the first.) Caregivers have a very difficult time dealing with patients who are up and wandering during the night.

Sometimes this wandering at night is accompanied by agitated behavior, called sundowning. It was once believed that sundowning occurred just at sunset when it began to get dark. More recent research indicates that sundowning behavior can occur any time of the day or night. Sundowning may result from fragmented sleep in older demented patients.

Much speculation has been done about the causes of sundowning. Dr. Donald Bliwise and others have proposed that this phenomenon may be related to changes in circadian rhythms since many of our rhythms become abnormal in dementia.

WHAT HAPPENS TO SLEEP IN PATIENTS LIVING IN NURSING HOMES?

Patients living in nursing homes have extremely fragmented sleep. Research from my laboratory showed that on average, patients in nurs-

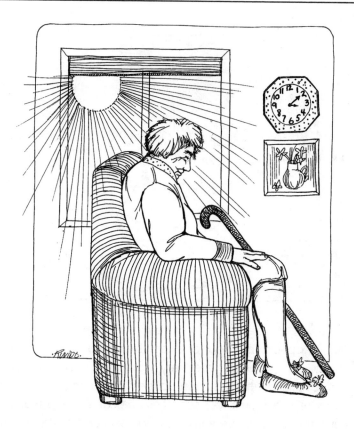

ing homes were never asleep for a full hour nor ever awake for a full hour, throughout the 24-hour day. In other words, these patients were constantly falling asleep and waking up all day and all night long.

Many factors contribute to this disturbed sleep. Chronic bed rest is common in nursing home patients, either because the patient is too sick to get out of bed, because of boredom, or because the staff had put the patient to bed early. Yet as described in Chapter 3, the longer an individual stays in bed, the more fragmented and disturbed sleep becomes. In addition, nursing home patients take multiple medications, all of which can contribute both to daytime sleepiness and to nighttime sleep disturbance. Sleep apnea is extremely common in this population—we found that 42% of the patients had

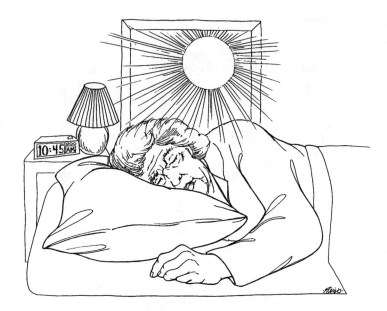

more than 5 apneas per hour of sleep. Dementia and sundowning, which also disrupt sleep, are very common in this population. Disturbed circadian rhythms, caused both by aging and by poor light exposure, contribute to poor sleep. (Recall that the majority of nursing home patients are almost never exposed to bright light.) Many patients nap because they are bored, and the consistent napping leads to disrupted sleep at night. It is the combination of all these problems that leads to the extremely fragmented sleep seen in this group of elderly patients.

CHAPTER SUMMARY

The belief about sleep and aging has always been that as we age, we need less sleep. We now know that the need for sleep does not change with age. Rather the ability to sleep decreases, and the ability to sleep is something you can learn.

12 DOCTORS, DRUGS, AND DEVICES

DOCTORS

When you feel that your nighttime sleep is so disturbed that you cannot function well during the day, it is time to see your doctor. Your doctor should try to determine the cause of your sleep disturbances. Depending on your problem, you may be referred to a sleep specialist.

The sleep specialist will usually begin by having you keep a sleep diary. This may be a form that you fill out every day for a week or two, or you might be asked to keep a small notebook. Your answers should be written down each morning, not at night before you go to bed, and certainly not in the middle of the night. The questions you most likely will be asked to answer include:

- What time did you go to bed last night?
- How long do you think it took you to fall asleep last night?
- How many times did you wake up during the night?
- How long did it take you to fall back to sleep?
- What time did you wake up in the morning?
- How did you feel when you woke up in the morning?

Some specialists may ask you to fill out the Stanford Sleepiness Scale (SSS) each morning. On the SSS, you rate how sleepy you feel when you wake up by choosing a number from 1 (feeling active and vital, alert, wide awake) to 7 (almost in a reverie; sleep onset soon; losing struggle to stay awake).

Stanford Sleepiness Scale

1. Feeling active and vital; alert, wide awake
2. Functioning at a high level, but not at peak; able to concentrate
3. Relaxed; awake, responsive, but not at full alertness
4. A little foggy; let down; not at peak
5. Foggy; slowed down; losing interest in staying awake
6. Sleepy; woozy; prefer to be lying down; fighting sleep
7. Almost in a reverie; sleep onset soon; losing struggle to stay awake

Other questions need to be filled out in the evening. These would include:

- How much caffeine did you consume today? What time was the last cup?
- How much alcohol did you drink today? What time did you last drink?
- What medications did you take today and at what times?
- Did anything stressful happen today?
- Did you take any naps today? How many and at what times?

The sleep diary will help both the sleep specialist and you determine what your normal sleep patterns are and what daytime activities might be affecting your sleep. You will be asked to bring the sleep diary with you to your first appointment.

In addition to the sleep diary, you may be sent a bed partner questionnaire. If you do not have a regular bed partner, this can be filled out by someone else living in your house or someone who visits frequently. The bed partner will be asked to describe your sleep habits both at night and during the day. The types of questions include:

- Does your bed partner snore?
- Do your bed partner's legs twitch, jerk, or kick during the night?

- Does your bed partner fall asleep during the day while:
  —watching television?
  —reading?
  —driving?
  —riding in a car or bus?
  —sitting with friends?

Whenever possible, your bed partner should accompany you to your first appointment.

During your first visit, the doctor may examine you and measure your blood pressure and your weight. However, most of the time will be spent talking to you about your sleep. The doctor will want to know:

- How long does it take you to fall asleep at night?
- How many times do you wake up during the night?
- Do you know what wakes you?
- Do you have difficulty falling back to sleep?
- Do you ever wake up at night short of breath or choking?
- Do you ever wake up at night confused?
- Are you aware of or have you been told that your legs twitch or jerk during the night?
- What time do you wake up in the morning?
- How do you feel when you wake up in the morning?
- Do you wake up with a headache in the morning?
- Are you aware of snoring, or have you been told that you snore?
- How loudly do you snore? Can your snoring be heard outside your bedroom?
- Are you aware of, or have you been told that you stop breathing at night?
- What position do you normally sleep in? Is your snoring worse in certain body positions? Is your snoring better in certain body positions?
- Do you ever feel paralyzed as you are falling asleep?

- Do you ever have vivid, frightening dreams as you are falling asleep?
- Are you sleepy during the day? Do you take naps on purpose? ("I'm tired, I think I'll lie down and take a nap.") How often and how long do you nap on purpose?
- Do you find yourself falling asleep without meaning to? Do you fall asleep reading, watching television, at meetings at work, while sitting with friends, at the movies?
- Have you ever had a near-miss automobile accident as a result of sleepiness?
- Have you ever had an automobile accident because of sleepiness?
- Do you ever experience episodes of weakness during the day?

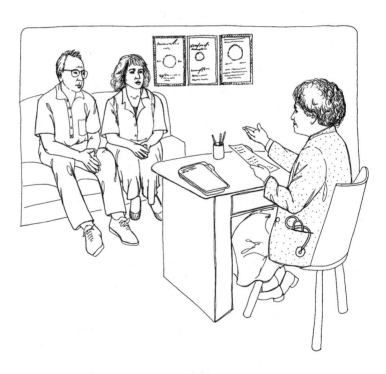

- How much alcohol do you drink? How often do you drink? What time of day do you drink?
- How much caffeine do you drink? How often do you drink? What time of day do you drink?
- Has your weight changed? Did your snoring and sleepiness get better, worse, or stay the same as your weight changed?
- What medications do you take? Do you ever take any sleeping pills or other medication to help you sleep?
- Does anyone in your family (your father, mother, brother, sister, etc.) snore or have other symptoms like yours?

If the doctor suspects sleep apnea, she will also look inside your mouth. Although your airway is open when you are awake, the doctor will look for signs of redness and enlarged structures (such as a long soft palate, a long uvula, a large tongue, or large tonsils). Sometimes special tests will need to be done to examine and take measurements of your airway.

DRUGS

The doctor will question you very carefully about all prescription and over-the-counter medications that you are taking. It is very helpful to write down all the names of the drugs you take regularly, as well as the amount and the time of day you take them.

All drugs have two names, the generic name (that is, the chemical name of the compound) and the trade or brand name. Sometimes, the same chemical compound might be made by more than one company and might therefore have more than one trade name. Generic names are never capitalized; trade names are always capitalized. You should write down the name of the medication as it appears on the medication container.

Almost all medications have the potential to affect your sleep, either by making it hard to sleep at night or by making you sleepy in the daytime. Having your physician adjust the time of day and the dose of your medications will sometimes improve your sleep complaint.

113

Common Drugs That Can Cause Insomnia

- Alcohol
- Beta blockers
- Bronchodilators
- Corticosteroids
- CNS Stimulants (for example caffeine, over-the-counter decongestants, theophylline, cocaine)

- Decongestants
- Diphenylhydantoin (Dilantin)
- Nicotine
- Stimulating antidepressants
- Thyroid hormones

Borrowed with permission from the National Sleep Foundation.

Antidepressants, drugs used to treat depression, often have an effect on nighttime sleep and daytime functioning. Of course, the amount that sleep is altered varies from drug to drug. In general, tricyclic antidepressants (such as amitriptyline [Elavil], doxepin [Sinequan], imipramine [Tofranil], or nortriptyline [Pamelor]) decrease the amount of REM sleep and might increase the amount of slow wave sleep. In addition, most cause some daytime sleepiness that could affect daytime performance. Other antidepressants (such as trazodone [Desyrel], fluoxetine [Prozac], or lithium) can also affect sleep. The amount of drug you take and the time of day you take it determines how the drug affects your sleep. For this reason, most doctors recommend that the more sedating drugs be taken at night. The use of monoamine oxidase inhibiting (MAOI) drugs (such as tranylcypromine [Parnate] or phenelzine [Nardil]), which are also used to treat depression, can result in fragmented, restless sleep with many awakenings and decreased amounts of REM sleep, as well as some daytime sleepiness.

Other drugs that are used to treat pulmonary disease, such as those used to treat asthma, affect sleep. Theophylline for example, can cause disturbed sleep because of its alerting properties. Drugs used to treat cardiovascular disease can also cause difficulty falling asleep and increased awakenings during the night.

114

Antidepressants Causing Sleepiness or Insomnia

Generic Name	Trade Name	Usual Dose
Antidepressants causing sleepiness		
amitriptyline	Elavil	100-300mg
desipramine	Norpramin	100-300mg
imipramine	Tofranil	100-300mg
nefazodone	Serzone	300-600mg
nortriptyline	Pamelor	50-150mg
sinequan	Doxepin	100-300mg
trazodone	Desyrel	200-400mg
Antidepressants causing insomnia		
bupropion	Wellbutrin	200-300mg
desipramine*	Norpramin	100-300mg
fluoxetine	Prozac	10-60mg
imipramine*	Tofranil	100-300mg
nortriptyline*	Pamelor	50-150mg
paroxetine	Paxil	10-50mg
sertraline	Zoloft	50-200mg
venlafaxine	Effexor	75-225mg

*These antidepressants can cause insomnia, as well as sleepiness, depending on the dose taken.

Antihistamines are used by many people to treat the common cold. Antihistamines also cause sleepiness. For this reason, many people use these drugs to help them sleep. However, there are no scientific studies to indicate that antihistamines help insomnia or prolong sleep during the night. It is easy to build up a tolerance to antihistamine (that is, the longer you take the antihistamine to help you sleep, the larger the dose you need for the drug to be effective). In addition, antihistamine causes daytime drowsiness.

Pain killers (analgesics) such as morphine will also make a person sleepy. People taking these drugs have impaired performance during the day and have decreased REM sleep at night. Aspirin,

115

Other Drugs That Can Cause Insomnia	
Generic Name	**Trade Name**
Cold, allergy, and asthmas drugs	
pseudoephedrine	Sudafed
theophylline	Theo-Dur
Gastrointestinal drugs	
cimetidine	Tagamet
Cardiovascular drugs	
methyldopa	Aldomet
hydrochlorothiazide	HydroDIURIL
propranolol	Inderal
furosemide	Lasix
quinidine	Quinidex
Neurologic drugs	
phenytoin	Dilantin

another pain killer, sometimes produces slight drowsiness and has been used by patients with insomnia to help them fall asleep. The sedating effect of aspirin is very mild and therefore it is not recommended to be used to help sleep.

Insomnia can also be caused by "recreational" drugs. Stimulants (amphetamines and cocaine) make it harder to fall asleep, reduce REM sleep, and disrupt sleep. During withdrawal, individuals can experience hypersomnia (excessive sleepiness) at first, followed by insomnia.

WHAT ABOUT SLEEPING PILLS?

Pharmacologic treatment should be aimed, whenever possible, at the underlying disorders, such as depression, anxiety disorder, pain, and so forth. Sleeping pills should be used for relief of symptoms and should not be used for more than a few weeks at a time.

Sleeping pills have four characteristics that need to be considered: dose (how much to take), rate of absorption (how long does it take the drug to become effective after you take it), half-life (how long it stays in the body), duration (how long to continue taking the drug). The half-life is important; drugs with long half-lives will still be in your system the next day and can cause side effects such as daytime sleepiness ("hangover"). Drugs with short half-lives are gone by morning, but may cause rebound insomnia if you stop taking them after a few nights. The physician, in deciding on the best sleeping pill to prescribe, must take into account your other medical diagnoses, age, your use of other medications, alcohol use, anticipated duration of treatment, and alternative forms of therapy. The physician should educate you, the patient, about the benefits and limitations of the chosen sleeping pill, its side effects, and appropriate use.

Patients should usually be prescribed low amounts of drug for short periods (2 to 3 weeks at most) and should be followed by visits or phone calls regularly if prescriptions are renewed. Treatment of insomnia should always aim at the lowest possible effective dose.

An ideal sleeping pill would be effective immediately, help you fall asleep faster, not affect the different levels of sleep but allow normal responses to things like the crying baby or the alarm clock. The ideal sleeping pill would leave no "hangover" (still feeling sleepy the next day) and you would not develop tolerance (begin to need larger and larger doses for it to be effective) or withdrawal effects when you stopped the pill. In addition, the pill would not affect breathing, memory, walking or coordination. Unfortunately, there is no such ideal substance.

All sleeping pills impair performance while in your body. However, sleeping pills with shorter half-lives, and therefore shorter duration of action, impair performance less the following day. A second side effect of sleeping pills is anterograde amnesia (amnesia for information obtained after the drug is ingested). Anterograde amnesia is a potential side effect of all hypnotics, but again, the dose and duration will determine the severity of the memory loss. In addition, sleep itself produces amnesia, therefore the interaction of the hyp-

117

notic and how fast an individual falls asleep will determine the amount of amnesia experienced. For example, people who fall asleep in under 7 minutes experience some amnesia; those falling asleep in 7 or more minutes experience no amnesia. The amnesia only becomes a problem when the individual needs to wake up during the night to perform a task (such as taking other medications), which he may later not remember. For most individuals sleeping at home this is not a problem.

Another problem associated with sleeping pills is that of rebound insomnia. Rebound insomnia occurs when the sleeping pill is suddenly stopped. Sleep gets worse for several nights, and the temptation is to begin taking the sleeping pill again. Rebound is also effected by dose and half-life. Hypnotics with short or intermediate half-lives are more likely to produce rebound insomnia. Some hypnotics with extremely short half-lives may even produce some rebound insomnia in the early morning hours. Those sleeping pills with longer half-lives self taper and therefore do not produce rebound. In addition, the higher the dose of the sleeping pill, the greater the chance of having rebound.

As with any medications, there are cautions and contraindications that need to be considered in the administration of sleeping pills. Sleeping pills should not be taken by patients with sleep-disordered breathing, women who are pregnant, drug abusers (particularly alcohol abusers), or by those individuals who may need to be alert during their sleep period (for example, physicians on call). In addition, caution should be used in prescribing sleeping pills to patients who snore loudly; who have renal, hepatic, or pulmonary disease; and who are elderly. Elderly patients should be prescribed the lowest possible dose because of decreases in metabolism and elimination rates.

Studies have shown that almost all sleeping pills, if given in adequate doses, help a person to fall asleep faster and stay asleep. The task for the physician is to determine the lowest adequate dose, that is, the dose that will promote sleep with the fewest side effects.

When and How Should Hypnotic Sleeping Pills be used

- Only when your physician prescribes them.
- For short-term insomnia, not longer than 2 to 3 weeks.
- Only intermittently (once every 2 to 3 nights) in chronic insomnia.
- At the lowest possible effective dose.

When Should Hypnotic Sleeping Pills be used with Caution

- When many other medications are being used.
- In elderly patients.
- In patients with certain medical problems such as renal impairment or severe pulmonary problems.
- In patients with psychiatric problems, such as depression.
- By people who need to be alert as soon as they wake up (such as physicians on call or firemen).
- In patients who snore loudly.

When Should Hypnotic Sleeping Pills not be Taken

- Without a doctor's prescription and without a proper diagnosis.
- For long time periods; that encourages dependence (psychologic addiction).
- With alcohol.
- When they produce daytime sleepiness.
- In pregnant women or nursing mothers.
- In patients with sleep disordered breathing.

Finally, no sleeping pill is recommended for chronic use. The appropriate administration is for acute, short-term use, and when necessary, in combination with behavioral therapy.

SOME OF THE MORE COMMONLY PRESCRIBED SLEEPING PILLS

Many classes of drugs are used as sleeping pills. Over the years these have included the benzodiazepines (such as Dalmane, Valium, Restoril, Halcion, Xanax, quazepam, estazolam, Ativan, ProSom), imidzopyridines (such as Ambien), chloral hydrate, antihistamines,

Generic Name	Trade Name	Available Dose	Rate of Absorption	Length of Action (Half-life)
Benzodiazepines				
estazolam	ProSom	1-2mg	fast	12-18 hours
flurazepam	Dalmane	7.5-30mg	fast	2-4 days
quazepam	Doral	7.5-15mg	fast	2-4 days
temazepam	Restoril	7.5-30mg	slow	10-20 hours
triazolam	Halcion	0.125-0.25mg	intermediate	2-5 hours
Imidzopyridine				
zolpidem	Ambien	5-10mg	intermediate	2-5 hours

some antidepressants (such as amitriptyline, doxepin and trazodone), barbiturates (such as Pentobarbital or Secobarbital; note that these drugs are extremely dangerous) and over-the-counter medications. The ones most commonly recommended and used for aiding sleep are some of the benzodiazepines and imidzopyridines because they are the safest sleeping aids available. Nevertheless, each drug varies in its chemical make up and side effects.

It is important for you and your doctor to determine which sleeping pill is best for you and for your type of sleeping problem.

WHAT ABOUT OVER-THE-COUNTER SLEEPING AIDS?

Over-the-counter (OTC) sleeping aids refer to those aids available without a doctor's prescription. Some common OTC sleeping aids are Sleep-Eze, Sominex, or Nytol. Most of these OTC aids contain anti-histamines that make you sleepy. Antihistamines may cause allergic reactions in some people and may interact negatively with other medications and with alcohol. Although these drugs may make you sleepy, they are not recommended for long-term use as sleeping aids.

DEVICES

Once your interview is complete, the doctor will decide if you need to have your sleep recorded. If you do, an appointment will be set for an evening that is convenient for you. You will be asked to come to the laboratory or clinic several hours before your normal bed time and you can be awakened at your chosen time in the morning.

When you arrive at the laboratory, you will first get ready for bed—put on your night clothes, brush your teeth and complete your normal nighttime routine. At that point you will be "wired up." You will have electrodes (sensors) placed on your scalp, around your eyes, and under your chin. These allow the determination of the different levels of sleep. Depending on what sleep disorder the doctor suspects, you may also have bands or wires around your chest to measure respiration, sensors under your nose to measure airflow, sensors on your chest to measure your heart rate, sensors on your legs to determine if you kick at night, and a small cylinder on your finger to measure the amount of oxygen in your blood. These wires and sensors are all noninvasive, that is, no skin is punctured. If additional information is required for other disturbances, additional wires and electrodes will be used.

Once all the wires are attached, you will lie down in bed. The wires are all long enough to allow you free movement—you can toss and turn if you would like to. If you need to get up during the night, you can call the technician over the intercom.

If you have sleep apnea, you may be tested with CPAP on the same night or on a second night (see Chapter 5). The mask used for the test will be fitted earlier in the evening before you go to bed. During the night, you will sleep with the mask, and different levels of pressure will be tested to determine which pressure is most appropriate for you.

In the morning, the wires will be removed and you will be free to leave. It can take several weeks for this type of record to be scored, but you will be contacted by the doctor with your results and with recommendations for treatment.

Sometimes, rather than record sleep in the laboratory, your doctor might suggest that your sleep be recorded in your own home. This is done with ambulatory monitoring, devices that allow you to walk about until you are ready to go to bed. Ambulatory monitors can record much of the same information that gets recorded in the laboratory, but obtain the information in a more natural environment, that is, your own bed. These devices are especially good for screening certain sleep disorders and for doing follow-up studies to test the effectiveness of your treatment.

Many of these portable devices have small computers that collect the physiologic information. You will be wired in the late after-

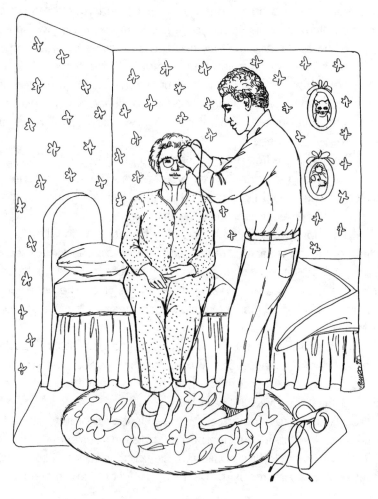

noon or evening in the laboratory or in your own home. The next morning, the technician will return to your home, or you will return to the clinic with the equipment. The data are then downloaded onto a large computer and scored for sleep and sleep problems.

Another type of portable recording device is the wrist actigraph. It has been shown that when we are awake, we tend to move our wrists, although when we are asleep we tend to be still. This observation has been translated into a device that measures wrist movement, and from that wrist movement, a doctor can distinguish wake from sleep. Actigraphs are small, watchlike devices that are worn on the wrist. Because of their electronics, these devices will record information for over a week, which allows physicians to gain information not only about night time behavior, but also about napping and daytime behavior. These recording devices are ideal for measuring sleep/wake patterns in patients with insomnia or circadian rhythm disturbances.

WHERE CAN I FIND OUT MORE INFORMATION ABOUT SLEEP SPECIALISTS AND SLEEP DISORDERS?

Many professional organizations deal with sleep and sleep disorders. The following annotated list provides the most current (as of publication of this book) name, address, phone number, and brief description of those organizations that supply information to the general public.

American Sleep Apnea Association (ASAA)
2025 Pennsylvania Ave, Suite 905
Washington, DC 20006
(202) 293-3650
Contact person: Christin Engelhardt

The purpose of the ASAA is to reduce disability associated with sleep apnea. Its audience is made up of sleep apnea patients. The ASAA is involved with public support groups for patients with sleep apnea, the AWAKE Network. There are approximately 100 AWAKE support groups in the United States.

123

American Sleep Disorders Association
1610 14th Street Northwest, Suite 300
Rochester, MN 55901-2200
(507) 287-6006

The membership of the American Sleep Disorders Association (ASDA) is made up of sleep disorders centers and of professional sleep clinicians and researchers. The purpose of this organization is to promote quality patient care and provide member services. The ASDA's main responsibilities include establishing standards of practice for the evaluation and treatment of sleep disorders and promoting education in sleep disorders medicine.

Better Sleep Council
333 Commerce Street
Alexandria, VA 22314
(703) 683-8371

The Better Sleep Council is a nonprofit organization dedicated to raising public awareness about the health benefits of sleep. Brochures and materials are available on request.

Narcolepsy Network
P.O. Box 1365
FDR Station
New York, NY 10150
(914) 834-2855

The Narcolepsy Network develops local chapters for patients with narcolepsy.

National Institutes of Health
National Center on Sleep Disorders Research
NIH/NHLBI/NCSDR
Two Rockledge Centre/Suite 7024
6701 Rockledge Dr. MSC 7920
Bethesda, MD 20892-7920
(301) 435-0199

The National Center on Sleep Disorders Research was established within the National Institutes of Health by the US Congress in 1993. The purpose of the center is to support research, research training, and dissemination of information about sleep disorders. The center also coordinates activities on sleep and sleep disorders among different agencies within the federal government, including the Departments of Health and Human Resources, Defense, and Transportation.

National Sleep Foundation
1367 Connecticut Avenue, NW
Suite 200
Washington, DC 20036
(202) 785-2300

The mission of the National Sleep Foundation (NSF) is to improve quality of life for the millions of Americans who suffer from sleep disorders, to prevent the catastrophic accidents that are related to poor or disorganized sleep, and to educate both professionals (physicians, nurses, etc.) and the public about sleep and sleep disorders. They publish newsletters and serve as a clearing house for information on sleep. The NSF can be contacted for information and brochures about any aspect of sleep or sleep disorders. The NSF can provide you with lists of accredited sleep centers in your city or state.

Narcolepsy and Sleep Disorders
P.O. Box 51113
Palo Alto, CA 94303-9559
(415) 424-8533

An international newsletter created for patients, physicians, and sleep researchers.

Restless Legs Syndrome Foundation (RLSF)
1904 Banbury Road
Raleigh, NC 27608

The purpose of the RLSF is to support patients with restless legs syndrome and their families. The membership is made up of patients with restless legs syndrome.

Sleep Disorders Dental Society
11676 Perry Hwy #1
Suite 1204
Wexford, PA 15090
(412) 935-0836

This organization is made up of dentists interested in the treatment of sleep disorders.

Society for Light Treatment and Biological Rhythms
10200 West 44th Ave, #304
Wheatridge, CO 80033
(303) 422-8894

The SLTBR can be contacted for information about circadian rhythms problems (such as jet lag or Seasonal Affective Disorder) or sleep disorders and light treatment.

ARE THERE OTHER BOOKS I CAN READ?

Carskadon, M: *Encyclopedia of sleep and dreaming*, 1993, New York, Macmillan.

Ferber, R: *Solve your child's sleep problems*, 1985, New York, Simon & Schuster.

GLOSSARY

Advanced Sleep Phase Syndrome People with advanced sleep phase syndrome complain of sleep maintenance insomnia; that is, they complain about waking up too early in the morning. These people generally get sleepy early in the evening, perhaps at 7:00 PM or 8:00 PM, and then wake up about eight hours later, at 4:00 AM or 5:00 AM. This is particularly common in older people.

Alpha Waves Brain waves produced when we are relaxed but awake, primarily in the frequency of 8 to 13 cycles per second.

Apnea Complete cessation of respiration.

Apnea Index The number of apneas (complete cessation of respiration) per hour of sleep. This number is used to help make the diagnosis of sleep apnea.

Beta Waves Brain waves produced when we are awake and alert, primarily in the frequency greater than 12 cycles per second.

Bruxism Tooth grinding during sleep.

Cataplexy One of the symptoms of Narcolepsy. It is a muscular weakness or paralysis usually brought on by strong emotions, such as anger, fear, strong laughter, or crying.

Central Sleep Apnea A type of sleep apnea caused when the respiratory centers in the brain briefly fail, causing a pause in respiration during sleep.

Circadian Rhythms Our internal, biologic rhythms that fluctuate approximately every 24 hours. The sleep/wake cycle is one example. Core body temperature and certain hormones also fluctuate.

Continuous Positive Airway Pressure (CPAP) The preferred treatment for sleep apnea. A comfortable nose mask is connected by a hose to a machine that blows air into the airway. The positive air pressure acts almost as a splint to keep the airway open during the night.

Delayed Sleep Phase Syndrome Often occurs in late adolescence, as our rhythms begin to phase delay. People with delayed sleep phase syndrome get sleepy later in the night, at about 1:00 AM or 2:00 AM and sleep until 10:00 AM or 11:00 AM. People with this syndrome are alert in the evening, but experience great sleepiness in the morning hours. Often these patients will complain of insomnia since they have great difficulty falling asleep at a more "traditional" time of the evening.

Delta Waves Brain waves produced during deep sleep, primarily in the frequency of less than 4 cycles per second.

Electroencephalogram (EEG) A measurement or recording of brain wave activity. Sensors are placed on the scalp and attached to a polygraph machine that can store and display the activity of the brain.

Electromyogram (EMG) Records muscle tension. Electrodes might be placed under the chin, on the legs, or wherever the sleep specialist needs to know about muscle tension.

Electrooculogram (EOG)   A tracing of eye movements. This is helpful in the identification of REM sleep.

Enuresis   Bed wetting. Described as a symptom, not as a disorder. It is defined as the inability to control urination during sleep. It usually occurs during the early hours of a child's sleep. By 6 years of age, most, but not all, children have learned control and are no longer wetting the bed.

Hypersomnia   Sleeping too much or being overly sleepy during the day. This symptom is also called excessive daytime sleepiness (EDS). Hypersomnia may be caused by many different factors, including not sleeping enough at night. It is important to discuss excessive daytime sleepiness with a doctor to determine if treatment, and which treatment, is necessary.

Hypnagogic Hallucinations   These are very vivid visual and auditory dreamlike phenomena that may occur in the patient who has narcolepsy, at the same time as sleep paralysis, that is, on falling asleep. The hallucinations are generally short-lived and end abruptly.

Hypnic Jerk   Also known as a sleep start, this is the feeling as you are falling asleep that you are falling, and you jerk yourself to stop your fall. This is normal and happens to everyone.

Hypopneas   Partial decrease in respiration.

Hypopnea Index   The number of hypopneas per hour of sleep.

Hypoventilation   This is breathing that is somewhat below normal in volume. Small decreases in breathing during sleep are common and normal. In some patients with lung disease or in obese patients, the normal small decreases in breathing that occur during sleep may result in decreases in oxygen levels in the blood and in severe cases, this can lead to heart problems.

Insomnia   A complaint of difficulty falling asleep, difficulty staying asleep, or both. Insomnia can be caused by medical problems, psychologic problems, drugs and medications, behavioral problems, circadian rhythm problems, or primary sleep disorders. Treatment of insomnia depends on the cause of the problem.

Maintenance of Wakefulness Test (MWT)   Measures how sleepy you are during the day. The patient is asked to sit in a dark room and to try to stay awake. Patients with excessive sleepiness have great difficultly staying awake in this situation.

Mixed Sleep Apnea   A type of sleep apnea generally beginning with a central component and followed by an obstructive component.

Multiple Sleep Latency Test (MSLT)   Measures how sleepy you are during the day. The patient is asked to go to sleep four to five times during the day, and the amount of time it takes to fall asleep is measured. Patients with sleep disorders characterized by excessive sleepiness generally fall asleep within 5 minutes.

Myoclonus Index   The number of leg jerks per hour of sleep. This number is used to help make the diagnosis of periodic limb movements in sleep.

Narcolepsy Sleep disorder characterized primarily by irresistible sleepiness during the day. In addition, patients with narcolepsy may experience cataplexy, sleep paralysis, and hypnagogic hallucinations.

Nightmares Frightening dreams that are usually very vivid and detailed. The content of the nightmare is frightening to the dreamer with common themes including being threatened, chased, hurt, or attacked. Nightmares occur during REM sleep.

Night Terrors Also called pavor nocturnus, these generally occur during sleep in the first third of the night. The person sits up in bed and screams. The episode can last several minutes, during which time the person experiences a racing heart, increased sweating, increased blood pressure, and dilated pupils. At the end of the episode, the person lies down and returns to normal sleep. If awakened, the person is confused for 15 to 30 minutes. There is no memory of the event in the morning.

Nocturnal Myoclonus See periodic limb movements in sleep.

Non–rapid Eye Movement (NREM) Sleep One of two states of sleep (see also REM sleep). NREM is subdivided into four stages of sleep. Stage 1 is the very lightest level of sleep and stage 4 is the deepest level of sleep. An individual spends 75% of the night in NREM sleep.

Obstructive Sleep Apnea A type of sleep apnea during which the muscles of the airway collapse, resulting in partial or complete blockage of airflow.

Parasomnias Intense, episodic physical events that occur during sleep or become worse during sleep. They occur primarily in children, but might be found in adults as well. Examples of parasomnias include sleepwalking, night terrors, bruxism, or sleeptalking.

Periodic Breathing Breathing in which the amount of respiration increases and decreases in a cyclic pattern (described as a crescendo and decrescendo pattern by musicians). It can occur while awake, but is frequently more noticeable and more severe during sleep. It is often associated with heart disease but can occur in normal subjects during the first few days at high altitudes.

Periodic Limb Movements in Sleep (PLMS) Also called nocturnal myoclonus, a condition in which the limbs (primarily the legs) twitch or jerk every 20 to 40 seconds during sleep. Most jerks cause brief awakenings and disrupt sleep.

Polygraph This is the machine that displays the biologic information as squiggly lines on a graph.

Polysomnograph The recording of biologic signals during sleep. The word comes from the Greek roots meaning: many (poly), sleep (somno), and graph (graphy).

Rapid Eye Movement (REM) Sleep One of two states of sleep (see also NREM sleep). Most of our dreaming takes place during REM sleep. During this state of sleep our bodies are paralyzed (except for our respiration and our eyes) to keep us from acting out our dreams.

Rapid Eye Movement (REM) Sleep Behavior Disorder Occurs when the muscle paralysis of REM sleep fails and the person experiences vigorous behavior during vivid dreaming. These behaviors, such as kicking, flailing, or punching, can result in injury both to the dreamer and the bed partner.

Restless Legs Syndrome (RLS) Associated with uncomfortable, creepy, crawling sensations in the lower legs, feet, or thighs, which result in an irresistible urge to move the limbs. These sensations generally occur when you are relaxed or resting and often interfere with falling asleep.

Respiratory Disturbance Index The number of apneas plus hypopneas per hour of sleep. This number is used to help make the diagnosis of sleep disordered breathing.

Sleep Apnea (Sleep Disordered Breathing) A disorder in which people stop breathing during sleep. The night is spent alternating between pausing in breathing, waking up, breathing, falling back to sleep, pausing in breathing, etc. Symptoms and consequences of sleep apnea can include, but are not limited to, loud snoring, daytime sleepiness, hypertension, heart irregularities, obesity, memory problems, and morning headaches.

Sleep Hygiene Means good sleep habits. Many people with sleep complaints have developed bad sleep habits over the years. Good sleep hygiene would include not spending too much time in bed; getting up at the same time each day; not looking at the clock in the middle of the night; avoiding caffeine, nicotine, and alcohol near bedtime; and exercising.

Sleep Paralysis A normal occurrence when an individual is waking up from REM sleep. Some patients experience sleep paralysis on falling asleep. Often sleep paralysis on falling asleep is a symptom of narcolepsy.

Sleeptalking Considered normal behavior that occurs most frequently in stage 2 sleep. There is no memory of this behavior, and it does not cause complaints of sleep disruption.

Sleepwalking Sleepwalkers are able to perform behaviors such as walking, opening doors, climbing up or down stairs, all while apparently sleeping. Sleepwalking generally occurs during the first third of the night.

Snoring Results from a partial narrowing of the airway caused by multiple factors such as inadequate muscle tone, large tonsils and adenoids, long soft palate, and limp tissue. About 25% of men and 15% of women are habitual snorers.

Theta Waves Brain waves produced during light sleep, primarily in the frequency of 4 to 7 cycles per second.

Zeitgebers Time cues that help synchronize circadian rhythms. Examples of zeitgebers include light or meals.

BIBLIOGRAPHY

Ancoli-Israel S, Kripke DF, Klauber MR et al: Sleep disordered breathing in community-dwelling elderly, *Sleep* 14(6):486-495, 1991.

Bliwise DL: Review: sleep in normal aging and dementia, *Sleep* 16:40-81, 1993.

Bootzin RR, Perlis ML: Nonpharmacologic treatments of insomnia, *J Clin Psychiatry* 53:37-41, 1992.

Campbell SS, Kripke DF, Gillin JC et al: Exposure to light in healthy elderly subjects and Alzheimer's patients, *Physiol Behav* 42:141-144, 1988.

Carskadon MA, editor: *Encyclopedia of sleep and dreaming*, New York, 1993, Macmillan.

Ferber R: *Solve your child's sleep problems*, New York, 1985, Simon & Schuster.

Hauri PJ: Consulting about insomnia: a method and some preliminary data, *Sleep* 16(4):344-350, 1993.

Hoddes E, Zarcone V, Smythe H et al: Quantification of sleepiness: a new approach, *Psychophysiology* 10(4):431-436, 1973.

Masand P, Popli AP, Weilburg JB: Sleepwalking, *Am Fam Physician* 51:649-654, 1995.

Morin CM: *Insomnia: psychological assessment and management*, New York, 1993, Guilord Press.

Spielman AJ, Saskin P, Thorpy MJ: Treatment of chronic insomnia by restriction of time in bed, *Sleep* 10:45-56, 1987.

Young T, Palta M, Dempsey J et al: Occurrence of sleep disordered breathing among middle-aged adults, *N Eng J Med* 328:1230-1235, 1993.

INDEX

A

Abnormal sleep, 14
Accidents, fatigue and, 31-32
Acetazolamide (Diamox) for sleep disordered breathing, 51
Activity
 brain, during sleep, 3
 physiologic, during sleep, 12-13
Adenoids, 40
Adolescents; see Teenagers
Advanced sleep phase syndrome, 74, 75
 symptoms of, 76
Age
 sleep apnea and, 44-45
 sleep cycles and, 12
 sleep phase changes and, 72, 74
Aging, sleep and, 101-108
Air pressure machine, 45-47
Airway, collapse of, during sleep, 36-38
Airway muscles, 36
Alcohol, 20-21
 narcolepsy and, 59
 and sleep disordered breathing, 43
Alcohol withdrawal, 98
Aldomet, effect on sleep of, 116
Allergies, enuresis and, 87
Alpha waves, 7
Alpha waves, aging and, 101-102
Alzheimer's disease, 106

Ambien, 119
Ambulatory sleep monitors, 121-123
American Sleep Apnea Association, 123
American Sleep Disorders Association, 124
Amitriptyline (Elavil), 27, 120
 effect on sleep of, 114
Amnesia, anterograde, from sleeping pills, 117-118
Amphetamines, effect on sleep of, 116
Amplitude of circadian rhythms, 69
Analgesics, effect on sleep of, 115-116
Anemia, 63
Anesthetics and sleep disordered breathing, 43
Anterograde amnesia from sleeping pills, 117-118
Antidepressants, 120
 effect on sleep of, 114, 115
 tricyclic, 27
  for cataplexy, 59
  PLMS aggravated by, 64
  for sleep disordered breathing, 51
Antihistamines, 119, 120
 effect on sleep of, 115
Anxiety
 in children and difficulty falling asleep, 84-85

Anxiety—cont'd
generalized, 28
Apnea, sleep; *see* Sleep apnea; Sleep disordered breathing
Apnea index, 35
Arthritis, 27, 63
rheumatoid, 65
ASAA (American Sleep Apnea Association), 123
ASDA (American Sleep Disorders Association), 124
Aspirin, 27
effect on sleep of, 115-116
Asthma, 28, 114
Ativan, 119
Auditory hallucinations, 54
AWAKE Network, 123
Awakening
during NREM sleep, 7, 9
regularity in time of, 18

B

Barbiturates, 120
Bed
curtail time in, 17-18
falling out of, 41
Bed partner questionnaire, 110-111
Bedroom clock, 19
Bedtime difficulties in children, 84-85
Bedwetting, 41, 86-88
treatment of, 87-88
Behavioral problems causing insomnia, 17
Behavioral treatments for insomnia, 23-27
Benzodiazepines, 27, 119, 120
for periodic limb movements in sleep, 66
for sleepwalking, 93
Beta waves, 6-7, 9
Better Sleep Council, 124
Biologic clocks, 4-5
aging and, 104-105

Bladder, small, causing enuresis, 86
Bladder control exercises for bedwetting, 88
Bliwise, Donald, 106
Blood, oxygen in, 6
Body rocking, 88-89
Body temperature
core, circadian rhythms in, 69, 70
drop in, 4-5
Bootzin, Richard, 24
Bradycardia, 41
Brain activity during sleep, 3
Brain waves
aging and, 101-102
during sleep, 5-6, 7
Brand name of drug, 113
Breathing
below normal, 38-39
deep, 23, 24
periodic, 38
during sleep, 6
sleep disordered, 35-51; *see also* Sleep disordered breathing
Breathing rates during sleep cycle, 12
Bright-light therapy, 74, 76
for jet lag, 78
for older people, 105
Bruxism, 98

C

Caffeine, 20
restless legs syndrome and, 65
Calculator, light exposure, to reduce jet lag, 78, 79
Campbell, Scott, 105
Cancer, 27
Cardiovascular disease, 114
Carskadon, Mary, 82
Cataplexy, 53-54, 56
treatment of, 59
Cataracts, 105
Central sleep apnea, 38
Chemical name of drug, 113

Children
    anxiety in, and difficulty falling
        asleep, 84-85
    sleep of, 81-89
    sleep complaints in, 85-86
    sleep needs of, 82-84
    sleep problems in, 2
Chin muscle tension during sleep, 5-6
Chloral hydrate, 119
Chocolate, caffeine in, 20
Chronic insomnia, 16
Chronic lung disease, 63
Chronic obstructive lung disease, 28
Cimetidine, effect on sleep of, 116
Circadian rhythms, 4-5, 18, 69-79
    aging and, 104-105
    disturbances of, 72
    measurement of, 69
    in nursing home patients, 108
Clitoral swelling during REM sleep, 13
Clocks in bedroom, 19
Clonazepam (Klonopin)
    for periodic limb movements in
        sleep, 66
    for REM sleep behavior disorder, 98
Cocaine, effect on sleep of, 116
Cognitive behavioral therapy, 26-27
Cole, Roger, 78
Congestive heart failure, 28, 45
Constipation causing enuresis, 86
Continuous positive airway pressure,
    45-47
Core body temperature, circadian
    rhythms in, 69, 70
Cough, chronic, 28
CPAP machine, 45-47
Cycles of sleep, 11
    aging and, 12

D

Dalmane, 119
Daytime sleepiness, 1, 31-33, 76; *see
    also* Narcolepsy
    excessive, 39

Deep breathing, 23, 24
Deep sleep, 7
Delayed sleep phase syndrome, 72,
    73
    symptoms of, 72, 74
Delta waves, 7
Dementia, 45, 98, 106
    in nursing home patients, 108
Dental devices, 50
Depression, 28
Desyrel, effect on sleep of, 114
Deviated septum, 38
Devices to record sleep, 120-123
Diabetes, 63, 104
    causing enuresis, 86
Diamox for sleep disordered breathing,
    51
Dilantin, effect on sleep of, 116
Disease; *see* specific disease
Doctors, 109-113
Dopaminergic drugs for periodic limb
        movements in sleep, 66
Doxepin (Sinequan), 120
    effect on sleep of, 114
Dozing, 7
DR2, narcolepsy and, 55
Dreaming, 7, 9
Dreams, frightening; *see* Nightmares
Drugs, 113-120
    effect on sleep of, 114
    hypersomnia caused by, 33
    insomnia and, 28-29
    and sleep disordered breathing,
        43
    for sleep disordered breathing, 51
Dry mouth on awakening, 41
Dysesthesias, 65
Dyskinesia, tardive, from L-dopa, 66

E

Elavil, effect on sleep of, 114
Electroencephalogram (EEG), 6
Electromyogram (EMG), 6
Electrooculogram (EOG), 6

Endocrine system activity during sleep, 13
Enuresis, nocturnal, 86-88
   treatment of, 87-88
Enuresis alarms, 88
Environment, sleeping, 22
Equipment to measure sleep activity, 5
Erections, penile, during REM sleep, 13
Estazolam, 119
Evening types, 71
Excessive daytime sleepiness (EDS), 31-33, 39
Exercise(s), 21
   bladder control, for bedwetting, 88
Eye movements during sleep, 5-6
   slow rolling, 7, 8

F

Falling out of bed, 41
Fatigue, accidents and, 31-32
Fears, nighttime, in children, 84-85, 86
Ferber, Richard, 85
Fibromyalgia, 27
Fluoxetine (Prozac)
   effect on sleep of, 114
   for sleep disordered breathing, 51
Foulkes, David, 95
Furosemide, effect on sleep of, 116

G

Gastrointestinal problems, 28
Generalized anxiety, 28
Generic name of drug, 113
Grinding teeth during sleep, 98
Growth hormone, 13

H

Halcion, 119
Hallucinations, hypnagogic, 54, 56
"Hangover" from sleeping pills, 117
Headaches, morning, 41
Headbanging, 88-89
Heart disease, 27, 40, 41, 104
   central sleep apnea and, 38

Heart failure, congestive, 28, 45
Heart irregularities in sleep apnea syndrome, 41
Heart rate, 6
   during sleep cycle, 12
Homeostatic regulation of sleep, 3
Hormones, 13
Hydrochlorothiazide, effect on sleep of, 116
HydroDiuril, effect on sleep of, 116
Hypersomnia, 31-33
   causes of, 31
   incidence of, 32
   treatment of, 33
Hypertension, 41, 45
   nocturnal, 42
Hyperthyroidism, enuresis and, 87
Hypnagogic hallucinations, 54, 56
Hypnic jerks, 61, 98
Hypnotic sleeping pills, indications and contraindications for, 119
Hypopneas, 35
Hypoventilation, 38-39

I

Imidzopyridines, 119, 120
Imipramine (Tofranil)
   for bedwetting, 87
   effect on sleep of, 114
Inderal, effect on sleep of, 116
Infant(s)
   sleep cycles of, 12
   sleep complaints in, 85-86
   sleep/wake patterns in, 81
Infections, urinary tract, causing enuresis, 86, 87
Insomnia, 6, 15-29
   antidepressants causing, 115
   behavioral treatments for, 23-27
   causes of, 16-22
   drugs causing, 28-29, 114, 116
   incidence of, 29
   medical problems causing, 27-28
   older people and, 102, 104

Insomnia—cont'd
    psychiatric problems causing,
        28
    psychophysiologic, 17
    rebound, 28
        from sleeping pills, 117, 118
    sleep maintenance, 76

J

Jerks, hypnic, 61, 98
Jet lag, 5, 70-71, 77-78

K

Kick, leg, in periodic limb movements
        in sleep, 62
    recording, 63
Kidney disease, 63
Kidney failure, 65
Klonopin
    for periodic limb movements in
        sleep, 66
    for REM sleep behavior disorder,
        98

L

"Larks," 71, 74
Laser assisted uvula-palatoplasty (LAUP),
        49
Lasix, effect on sleep of, 116
L-dopa for periodic limb movements in
        sleep, 66
Leg kick in periodic limb movements in
        sleep, 62
    recording, 63
Leukemia, 63
Light exposure calculator to reduce jet
        lag, 78, 79
Limb movements during sleep, 6
    periodic, 61-67
Lithium, effect on sleep of, 114
Lunch, sleepiness after, 4
Lung disease, 27, 28, 104
    chronic, 63

M

Maintenance of wakefulness test, 58
Measurement, sleep, 5-6
Medical problems causing insomnia,
        27-28
Medications; *see* Drugs
Melatonin, 13, 79
Menopause, 105-106
Methyldopa, effect on sleep of, 116
Mild sleep apnea, treatment of, 49-50
Mixed sleep apnea, 38
Monoamine oxidase inhibiting (MAOI)
            drugs, effect on sleep of, 114
Morin, Charles, 26
Morning headaches, 41
Morning stiffness, 27
Morning types, 71
Morphine
    effect on sleep of, 115
    and sleep disordered breathing, 43
Mouth, dry, on awakening, 41
Movement(s)
    excessive, during night, 41
    eye, during sleep, 5-6
    limb, during sleep, 6
    periodic, 61-67
Multiple sclerosis, 98
Multiple sleep latency test, 57-58
Muscle tension during sleep, 5-6, 12
Muscles, airway, 36
Myoclonus, nocturnal; *see* Periodic limb
            movements in sleep
Myoclonus index, 63

N

Names of drugs, 113
Napping
    for narcolepsy, 53, 59
    in nursing home patients, 107, 108
Narcolepsy, 53-59
    causes of, 55-56
    diagnosis of, 57-58
    incidence of, 57
    treatment of, 59

Narcolepsy Network, 124
Narcolepsy and Sleep Disorders, 125
Narcolepsy tetrad, 53, 54
Narcotics and sleep disordered breathing, 43
Nardil, effect on sleep of, 114
Nasal passages, blocked, 38
National Center on Sleep Disorders Research, 124
National Foundation for Sleep and Related Disorders in Children, 124
National Institutes of Health, National Center on Sleep Disorders Research, 124
National Sleep Foundation, 125
Need for sleep, 14
Neurologic disease, central sleep apnea and, 38
Newsletters about sleep, 125
Nicotine, 20
Night, working at, 76-77
Night terrors, 93-95
    nightmares versus, 95-96
    treatment of, 96-97
Nightmares, 95
    night terrors versus, 95-96
    treatment of, 96-97
Nighttime fears in children, 84-85, 86
Nocturia, 104
Nocturnal enuresis, 86-88
    treatment of, 87-88
Nocturnal hypertension, 42
Nocturnal myoclonus; *see* Periodic limb movements in sleep
Non-rapid eye movement sleep, 7, 11
    awakening during, 7, 9
    narcolepsy and, 56-57
    physiologic activity during, 12-13
Normal sleep, 6-10
Nortriptyline (Pamelor), effect on sleep of, 114
NREM sleep; *see* Non-rapid eye movement sleep

NSF (National Sleep Foundation), 125
Nucleus, suprachiasmatic, 4
    and circadian rhythms, 69
Nursing home patients, sleep in, 106-108
Nytol, 120

O

Obesity, 45
Obstructive lung disease, chronic, 28
Obstructive sleep apnea, 36-38, 41
Older people
    insomnia in, 102, 104
    normal changes in sleep in, 101-102
    in nursing homes, sleep in, 106-108
    periodic limb movements in sleep in, 105
    sleep and, 101
    sleep disordered breathing in, 105
Opiates for periodic limb movements in sleep, 66
Osteoarthritis, 27
Over-the-counter sleeping aids, 120
Overweight and sleep disordered breathing, 40
"Owls," 71, 72
Oxygen in blood, 6

P

Pain
    chronic, 104
    causing insomnia, 27
Pain killers
    effect on sleep of, 115-116
    for periodic limb movements in sleep, 65, 66
Palate, soft, 36
Pamelor, effect on sleep of, 114
Paradoxic sleep, 9
Paralysis, sleep, 12, 54, 56
Parasomnias, 91-99
Parent, sleep problem in, 2

Paresthesias, 65
Parkinson's disease, 98
    drugs for, for periodic limb move-
        ments in sleep, 66
Parnate, effect on sleep of, 114
Patients, nursing home, sleep in, 106-
    108
Pavor nocturnus, 93
Penile erections during REM sleep, 13
Pentobarbital, 120
Periodic breathing, 38
Periodic limb movements in sleep, 61-
    67
    aging and, 105
    causes of, 65
    diagnosis of, 63-64
    treatment of, 65-66
Pharynx, 36, 38
Phase of circadian rhythms, 69
Phase-advancement, 70
Phase-delay, 70
Phasic sleep behaviors, 13
Phenelzine (Nardil), effect on sleep of,
    114
Phenytoin, effect on sleep of, 116
Physiologic activity during sleep, 12-13
Physiology of sleep, 6-7
"Pins and needles" sensations in legs,
    65
Polygraph, 6
Polysomnography, 6
Position, changing, for sleep apnea,
    50
Postprandial dip, 4
Preadolescents, sleep needs of, 82
Pregnancy, 65
Progressive relaxation training, 23
Prolactin, 13
Propranolol, effect on sleep of, 116
ProSom, 119
Protriptyline (Vivactil) for sleep disor-
        dered breathing, 51
Prozac
    effect on sleep of, 114

Prozac—cont'd
    for sleep disordered breathing, 51
Pseudoephedrine, effect on sleep of,
    116
Psychiatric problems causing insomnia,
    28
Psychophysiologic insomnia, 17
Pulmonary disease, 27, 28, 114

Q

Quazepam, 119
Quindex, effect on sleep of, 116
Quinidine, effect on sleep of, 116

R

Rapid eye movement sleep, 7, 9, 10,
    12
    narcolepsy and, 56-57
    physiologic activity during, 12-13
    tonic and phasic behaviors during,
        13
Rapid eye movement sleep behavior
        disorder, 97-98
Rebound insomnia, 28, 117, 118
Reflux, gastrointestinal, 28
Relaxation training, progressive, 23
REM sleep; see Rapid eye movement
        sleep
REM sleep behavior disorder, 97-98
Renal disease, 63
Respiratory disturbance index (RDI),
    35
Restless legs syndrome, 65
Restless Legs Syndrome Foundation,
    125
Restoril, 119
    for periodic limb movements in
        sleep, 66
Rheumatoid arthritis, 65
Rheumatologic problems, 27
Rhythms, circadian; see Circadian
        rhythms
Rocking, body, 88-89
Rotating work schedules, 76-77

S

Savage, Henry, 78
Sclerosis, multiple, 98
Screaming from night terrors, 93-94;
    see also Night terrors
Secobarbital, 120
Septum, deviated, 38
Shift work problems, 76-77
Siestas, 4
Sinemet for periodic limb movements in
    sleep, 66
Sinequan, effect on sleep of, 114
Sleep
    abnormal, 14
    aging and, 101-108
    assessment of problems with, 111-
        113
    of children, 81-89
    devices to record, 120-123
    fragmented, in nursing home
        patients, 106-108
    homeostatic regulation of, 3
    measurement of, 5-6
    need for, 14
        in children, 82-84
    non-rapid eye movement (NREM),
        7, 11
        awakening during, 7, 9
        narcolepsy and, 56-57
        physiologic activity during, 12-
            13
    periodic limb movements in, 61-67;
        see also Periodic limb move-
        ments in sleep
    problems with, 1-2
    purpose of, 3
    rapid eye movement (REM), 7, 9,
        10, 12
        narcolepsy and, 56-57
        physiologic activity during, 12-13
        tonic and phasic behaviors dur-
            ing, 13
    stages of, 7, 11-12
    types of, 6-10

Sleep apnea, 35-51; see also Sleep
        disordered breathing
    age and, 44-45
    central, 38
    enuresis and, 87
    mild, treatment of, 49-50
    mixed, 38
    in nursing home patients, 107-108
    obstructive, 36-38
    physical signs suggestive of, 113
Sleep apnea syndrome, 35, 41; see
        also Sleep disordered
        breathing
Sleep architecture, 11
    aging and, 102
Sleep behavior disorder, rapid eye
        movement, 97-98
Sleep complaints in infants and chil-
        dren, 85-86
Sleep cycle, aging and, 102
Sleep deprivation, 3
Sleep diary, 109, 110
Sleep disorders, sources of information
        about, 123-126
Sleep Disorders Dental Society, 125
Sleep efficiency, aging and, 102
Sleep hygiene
    good, rules for, 17-23
    poor, 17
Sleep laboratory, 120-123
Sleep maintenance insomnia, 76
Sleep monitors, 120-123
    ambulatory, 121-123
Sleep paralysis, 12, 54, 56
Sleep restriction therapy, 25-26
Sleep specialist, 109-113
    sources of information about, 124-
        125
Sleep spindles, 7
Sleep starts; see Hypnic jerks
Sleep disordered breathing, 35-51
    aging and, 105
    causes of, 36-39
    incidence of, 44-45

Sleep disordered breathing—cont'd
symptoms of, 39-42
testing for, 43
treatment of, 45-51
Sleep-Eze, 120
Sleep/wake patterns in infants, 81;
see also Circadian rhythms
Sleepiness
antidepressants causing, 115
daytime, 1, 31-33, 76; see also
Narcolepsy
excessive, 39
excessive, 6
Sleeping aids, over-the-counter, 120
Sleeping environment, 22
"Sleeping in," 18
Sleeping pills, 116-119
commonly prescribed, 119-120
hypnotic, indications and contraindi-
cations for, 119
causing insomnia, 28
for periodic limb movements in
sleep, 65, 66
and sleep disordered breathing, 42-
43
Sleeptalking, 99
Sleepwalking, 91-93
treatment of, 93
Slow rolling eye movements, 7, 8
Slow wave sleep, 7
Snack before bedtime, 21-22
Snoring, 2, 36, 37, 38, 39-40
treatment of, 45, 47, 49
Society for Light Treatment and
Biological Rhythms, 125-126
Soda, caffeine in, 20
Soft palate, 36, 40
Sominex, 120
Spielman, Arthur, 24
Stage 1 sleep, 7, 8, 11
Stage 2 sleep, 7, 11
Stage 3 sleep, 7, 11
Stage 4 sleep, 7, 11
Stanford Sleepiness Scale (SSS), 109-
110

Steroids secreted during sleep, 13
Stiffness, morning, 27
Stimulants, effect on sleep of, 116
Stimulus-control therapy, 24-25
Stomach problems, 104
Stress, enuresis and, 87
Stroke, 40
Sudafed, effect on sleep of, 116
Sundowning, 106
in nursing home patients, 108
Suprachiasmatic nucleus, 4
and circadian rhythms, 69
Surgery
for sleep apnea, 47-49
for snoring, 47, 49

T

Tachycardia, 41
Tagamet, effect on sleep of, 116
Talking in sleep, 99
Tardive dyskinesia from L-dopa, 66
Tau of circadian rhythms, 69
Teenagers
phase-delay in, 72
sleep needs of, 82
Temazepam (Restoril) for periodic limb
movements in sleep, 66
Temperature, body
core, circadian rhythms in, 69, 70
drop in, 4-5
Temperature regulation during sleep
cycle, 12
Tension, chin muscle, during sleep, 5-6
Terrors, night, 93-95
nightmares versus, 95-96
treatment of, 96-97
Test
maintenance of wakefulness, 58
multiple sleep latency, 57-58
Theo-24 for sleep disordered breathing,
51
Theo-Dur
effect on sleep of, 116
for sleep disordered breathing, 51

Theophylline (Theo-Dur, Theo-24)
  effect on sleep of, 114, 116
  for sleep disordered breathing, 51
Theta waves, 7
Thyroid hormone, 13
Tobacco, 20
Tofranil, effect on sleep of, 114
Tongue, 36, 38
Tonic sleep behaviors, 13
Tonsils, 36, 38, 40
Tooth grinding, 98
Trade name of drug, 113
Traffic accidents, 32
Transient insomnia, 15-16
Tranylcypromine (Parnate), effect on
  sleep of, 114
Trazadone, 120
Trazodone (Desyrel), 120
  effect on sleep of, 114
Tricyclic antidepressants, 27
  for cataplexy, 59
  effect on sleep of, 114
  PLMS aggravated by, 64
  for sleep disordered breathing, 51
Tryptophan, 21-22
Tylenol with codeine for periodic limb
  movements in sleep, 66

U
Ulcers, 104
Uremia, 63, 65
Urinary tract infections causing enuresis,
  86, 87
Urologic problems causing enuresis, 86
Uvula, 36, 38
Uvula-palatoplasty, laser assisted, 49
Uvulopalatopharyngoplasty (UPPP), 47-
  48

V
Vaginal swelling during REM sleep, 13
Valium, 119
Vascular disorders, 98
Vivactil for sleep disordered breathing,
  51

W
Wandering at night, 106
Weakness from cataplexy, 54
Weight gain and sleep disordered
  breathing, 40
Weight loss for sleep apnea, 49
Withdrawal, alcohol, 98
Working at night, 76-77
Worry, 22

X
Xanax, 119

Y
Young, Terry, 44

Z
Zeitgebers, 69-70